Answering Patients' Questions About Vascular Medicine

Susanne Regus

Answering Patients' Questions About Vascular Medicine

170 Patient-Friendly Explanations

Springer

Susanne Regus
Abteilung für Gefäßchirurgie
Universitätsklinikum Regensburg
Regensburg, Germany

ISBN 978-3-662-72770-6 ISBN 978-3-662-72771-3 (eBook)
https://doi.org/10.1007/978-3-662-72771-3

Translation from the German language edition: "Patientenfragen zur Gefäßmedizin beantworten" by Susanne Regus, © Der/die Herausgeber bzw. der/die Autor(en), exklusiv lizenziert an Springer-Verlag GmbH, DE, ein Teil von Springer Nature 2025. Published by Springer Berlin Heidelberg. All Rights Reserved.

This book is a translation of the original German edition "Patientenfragen zur Gefäßmedizin beantworten" by Susanne Regus, published by Springer-Verlag GmbH, DE in 2025. The translation was done with the help of an artificial intelligence machine translation tool. A subsequent human revision was done primarily in terms of content, so that the book will read stylistically differently from a conventional translation. Springer Nature works continuously to further the development of tools for the production of books and on the related technologies to support the authors.

This Springer imprint is published by the registered company Springer-Verlag GmbH, DE, part of Springer Nature.
The registered company address is: Heidelberger Platz 3, 14197 Berlin, Germany

Preface

This book is intended for readers who, as physicians or nurses, regularly inform and advise patients or their relatives about vascular medical diseases, their causes, and treatment options. Here, they will find easily understandable answers to the most common questions, which they can pass on to concerned or interested medical laypersons.

In the course of my many years working as a hospital physician specializing in vascular surgery, I have been asked numerous questions by patients about their illnesses. I was repeatedly surprised at how difficult it can sometimes be to explain the causes and treatment options of their condition to patients and their relatives in a way that is easily understandable to laypeople.

The patient's understanding of their illness and the available treatment options is a crucial component for successful therapy. Therefore, in addition to optimal hospital care—from outpatient preparation through inpatient admission, surgery, and aftercare—special attention should be given to personal, "eye-level" conversations to answer all patient questions in a comprehensible and empathetic manner.

Below is an overview of common, as well as rarer, vascular surgical conditions. This is followed by answers to frequently asked questions posed by patients with vascular surgical diseases. The answers are formulated in layman's terms, with a focus on everyday clinical experience rather than scientific studies. Patients do not need any medical knowledge to understand the answers. Technical terms are rarely used, and when they are, they are explained and replaced with colloquial expressions.

This book aims to help bridge the gap between stress, hectic routines, and "medical jargon" in everyday clinical practice on the one hand, and the questions, concerns, and needs of patients on the other.

I hope that this book will help as many patients as possible to understand their illness, so that they can work together with their treating physicians to choose the optimal therapeutic approach.

Regensburg
Germany

Prof. Dr. med. Susanne Regus

Conflict of Interest The author has no conflicts of interest relevant to the content of this manuscript.

Contents

What Do Vascular Specialists Actually Do?

When Should You Actually See a Vascular Surgeon?
Vascular surgeons treat all vessels from the neck to the foot, except for vessels in the head, the heart, and the initial part of the main artery, the so-called aortic arch. I have deliberately left out the head, as other specialists, namely neurosurgeons, are responsible here. Cardiologists and cardiac surgeons are responsible for the heart.

Peripheral Arterial Occlusive Disease (PAOD)
Vascular surgeons treat **narrowed arteries** in the so-called peripheral arterial occlusive disease, usually abbreviated as **PAOD**. This is also known as **intermittent claudication** or "window shopper's disease," because poor blood flow to the legs means only short distances can be walked. After brief stops, for example in front of shop windows, walking can be resumed, which is where the name comes from. The pain often occurs in the calves while walking and disappears again at rest (see Fig. 1).

By dilating vessels or creating bypasses, blood flow to the leg can be improved. This then makes it possible to walk longer distances without pain.

"The Open Leg"
Chronic wounds that do not heal due to poor blood circulation are also a typical sign of PAOD. By creating a bypass, which is performed by the vascular surgeon, wounds can heal more quickly and the risk of amputation is greatly reduced.

Amputations may still be necessary, however, if the infection is so advanced that the leg can no longer be saved and there is also a risk of sepsis. In such critical situations, the patient's life is more important than the limb ("life before limb"), and the only option left for the vascular surgeon is to remove the leg so that the patient does not die from sepsis.

S. Regus, *Answering Patients' Questions About Vascular Medicine*,
https://doi.org/10.1007/978-3-662-72771-3_1

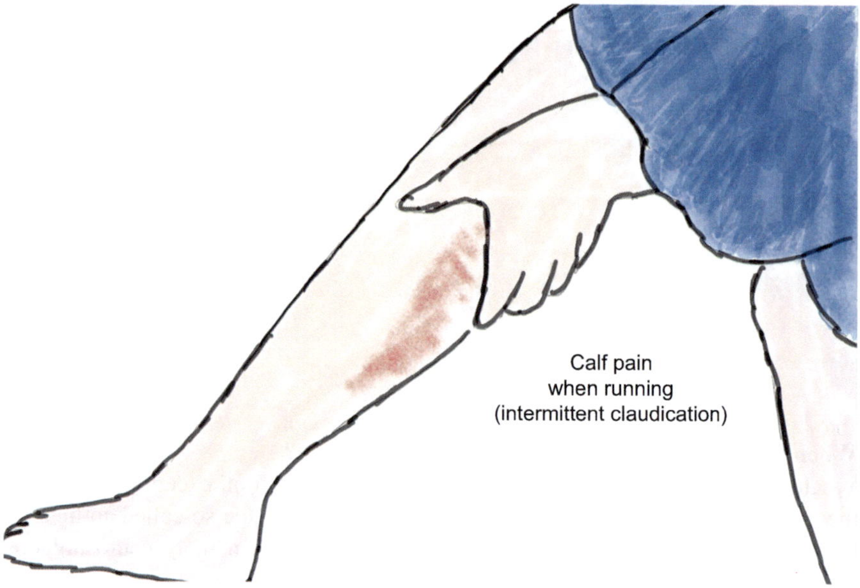

Fig. 1 Typical location of calf pain in "window shopper's disease"

Diabetes and Blood Vessels

People who suffer from "diabetes," so-called **diabetics,** have an increased risk of developing vascular diseases and tend to develop wounds and infections on the foot. Sometimes minor surgical procedures are sufficient to clean the wounds and promote healing. However, bypass surgery to bridge vascular occlusions is often necessary here as well.

"Cold Leg"

Acute **vascular occlusion** is also part of the field of vascular surgery and is highly feared. "Acute" means that the occlusion occurs suddenly and abruptly, "out of the blue," and is very painful. Doctors often refer to it as a "cold leg," describing the typical symptom: in addition to pain, there is a pronounced sensation of cold.

Stroke

Not only the arteries of the legs and arms (extremities) are treated by vascular surgeons, but also the **carotid arteries.** This may be necessary in patients who have already suffered a stroke. But even in asymptomatic patients with increasing narrowing of the carotid artery, surgery is recommended once a certain degree of stenosis is reached. In these cases, the aim is to prevent a **stroke**.

Aneurysms of the Aorta

Arteries can not only become too narrow, but also too wide. These pathological **dilations** (medically called **aneurysms**) are treated by vascular surgeons once they reach a certain diameter, in order to prevent **rupture (bursting)**. The larger the diameter of an aneurysm, the higher the risk of rupture. A rupture that has already occurred is a very dangerous situation that, if left untreated, leads to **death from bleeding**. The most commonly affected vessel is the main artery (aorta) in the chest and abdomen.

Dialysis

Patients with kidney disease who require **dialysis** need a well-accessible vascular access, which is medically referred to as a **shunt**. Creating a shunt is a classic vascular surgical procedure. However, many **shunt operations** are now performed on an outpatient basis without a hospital stay.

Vascular Injuries

Vascular injuries after accidents (trauma), so-called traumatic vascular lesions, typically occur in previously healthy vessels. The cause may be sharp objects or bone fragments in the case of a complicated fracture. Since these injuries often lead to significant bleeding, they usually need to be sutured as an emergency and sometimes replaced. This too falls within the scope of vascular surgery.

Vascular Diseases in Athletes

Vascular diseases caused by too much **exercise** or strain at **work** are very rare. As a rule, sports and physical activity are healthy for the vessels. Nevertheless, overuse from repetitive rapid movements, for example in professional cycling, can lead to **thickening** of the vessel wall and ultimately to narrowing. In these cases as well, vascular surgeons are the first point of contact.

Varicose Veins

Venous diseases are common vascular diseases, but they affect not the high-pressure (arterial) but the so-called low-pressure system. These include **thromboses** and **varicose veins**, which are generally not life-threatening conditions. Varicose veins, medically referred to as varices, are dilations of the superficial veins, mostly in the leg. In thrombosis, on the other hand, clots form in the veins, and here too the legs are most often affected. However, thromboses occur more frequently in the deep veins, which are not visible from the outside.

Venous Thromboses

Severe bleeding complications, as seen with arteries, do not occur in veins; however, in venous thrombosis, clots can travel to the lungs, which is a feared complication known as pulmonary embolism.

Arteriosclerosis

1. ***Is atherosclerosis really more dangerous than a tumor?***

For many years, vascular diseases have been the number one cause of death in industrialized countries, even ahead of malignant tumors. Since the vast majority of vascular diseases are due to atherosclerosis in the form of vascular calcification and fatty deposits, it is unfortunately true that atherosclerosis is a serious disease and has now overtaken cancer in terms of fatal outcomes. Important examples of dangerous and sometimes fatal vascular diseases include heart attacks, strokes, and rupture of the aorta. Atherosclerosis is preventable, and everyone can (and should!) do something to prevent it from occurring or to reduce its severity. This is where atherosclerosis and cancer differ, as the latter often represents a fateful disease without patient influence. This makes it all the more important to be aware of vascular diseases and their risk factors, which is the purpose of the following explanations and information on this topic.

2. ***What does arteriosclerosis literally mean?***

The term **arteriosclerosis** refers to all diseases that lead to calcification, hardening, and narrowing of arteries. **"Arterio-"** stands for arteries, also called arteriën in medical terminology. The term **"sclerosis"** is the technical term for hardening.

3. ***Are there different forms of vascular calcification?***

Arteriosclerosis is an umbrella term for all types of vascular calcification and hardening. Depending on the nature of the deposits and the underlying disease, arteriosclerosis is divided into three subtypes:

1. Arteriolosclerosis
2. Mediasclerosis
3. Atherosclerosis

S. Regus, *Answering Patients' Questions About Vascular Medicine*,
https://doi.org/10.1007/978-3-662-72771-3_2

4. ***Is it important to know these subtypes?***

Since **atherosclerosis** is the most common of the three subtypes, the terms atherosclerosis and arteriosclerosis are often used interchangeably, both in everyday language and by many physicians. Therefore, **atherosclerosis** is certainly the most important subtype of **arteriosclerosis**, and its name is one you should be familiar with.

Nevertheless, I would like to briefly discuss the individual subtypes of arteriosclerosis.

5. ***What is meant by arteriolosclerosis?***

In **arteriolosclerosis**, deposits form in the walls of smaller arteries, such as those in the fingers, toes, or kidneys. However, these deposits do not consist of lipids (fat), but of so-called hyaline membranes. In terms of consistency, these are comparable to soft plastic and are usually colorless and translucent. They arise mainly as a result of poorly controlled high blood pressure or as a consequence of diabetes mellitus. In medical terminology, the suffix **"-lo"** is often used to denote smaller structures; it can be considered a diminutive form. Thus, **arteriolo-** is the "diminutive" of **arterio-** and refers to small arteries.

6. ***What exactly is mediasclerosis?***

In **mediasclerosis**, which is also called **Mönckeberg sclerosis** after its first describer, there is a circular (i.e., affecting the entire circumference of the artery) calcification and hardening of the muscular layer of medium-sized and small arteries. The muscular layer lies between the inner layer (intima) and the outer layer (adventitia), and thus represents the middle layer of the vessel wall. This is where the term **"media"** comes from, which is equivalent to **middle**. In both arteriolosclerosis and atherosclerosis, it is always the inner layer (intima) that is affected. Mediasclerosis is most commonly found in the lower leg or foot, with diabetes mellitus being the main risk factor in its development.

7. ***What is special about atherosclerosis?***

In **atherosclerosis**, the most common and important form of arteriosclerosis, deposits of fat, cholesterol, and calcium form in the **inner layer (intima)** of arteries. These deposits are also called plaques. These deposits cause hardening **(sclerosis)** of the arterial wall. The term **"athero"** was chosen in reference to **atheromas**. These are nodular deposits in the skin around sebaceous glands, which appear like large **blackheads** ("pimples"). Since the contents of **atherosclerotic** plaques look similar to those of atheromas in the skin, atherosclerosis was given this name when it was first described. In contrast to atheromas, which arise from secretions of sebaceous glands, atherosclerotic plaques are formed by cholesterol crystals and fats from the bloodstream depositing in the vessel wall. The more fat and cholesterol accumulate in the arterial wall, the greater the narrowing becomes. In extreme cases, a complete blockage can occur.

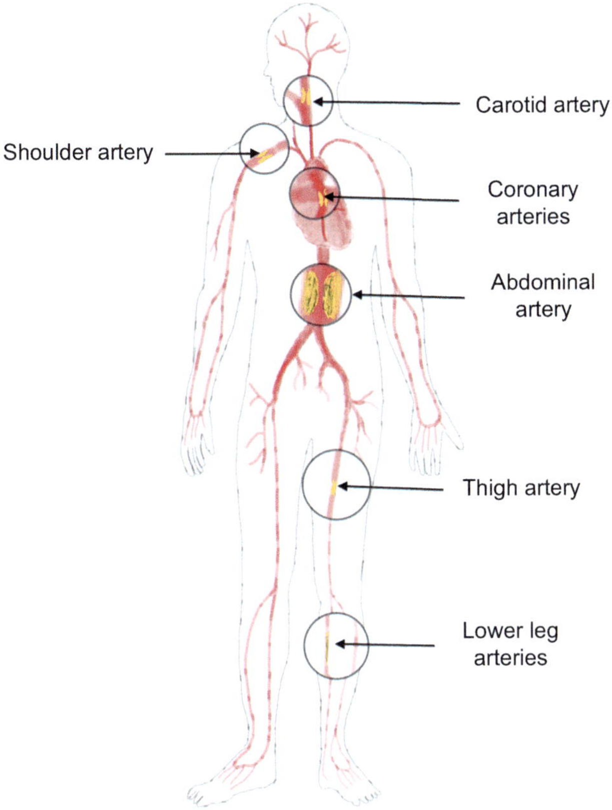

Fig. 1 Vascular regions frequently affected by atherosclerosis

Since all arteries in our body, from head to toe and from large to small, can be affected by atherosclerosis, the problems and symptoms are highly variable (see Fig. 1).

8. ***It is said that vascular calcification is a widespread disease. Is that true?***

Atherosclerosis is referred to as a widespread disease, and this is not without reason. It is a so-called degenerative disease, which means it is a type of "age-related disease" and a sign of wear and tear. Therefore, it is not surprising that the risk of developing the disease increases with age:

AGE	AFFECTED INDIVIDUALS
Young people up to the ***age of 40***	< 1 %
Among those ***aged 40 to 50*** already about	2 %
Among those ***aged 50 to 60*** already	5 %

AGE	AFFECTED INDIVIDUALS
Among ***60- to 70-year-olds*** every 10th person, that is	10 %
Among ***70- to 80-year-olds***	15 %
From age 80 about every 5th person, that is	20 %

Please do not be alarmed, even if you are already a bit older and have not had any problems with your arteries so far. You may now be thinking that you must also have vascular calcification. Of course, it is possible, but in many cases, and especially if you have no symptoms, you should not be worried or even afraid. Vascular calcification in advanced age is considered completely normal from a medical perspective and does not necessarily have clinical significance.

9. ***Roughly how high is the risk of developing atherosclerosis over the course of a lifetime?***

This cannot be answered in general terms, but the risk is about 10%, meaning that, roughly estimated, in industrialized countries every 10th person will experience a complication from vascular calcification during their lifetime.

In developing countries as well as in European countries with a primarily Mediterranean diet, the risk of disease is significantly lower, which is attributed, among other things, to the protective effect of fresh vegetables, fruit, and unsaturated fatty acids (such as olive oil).

10. ***How does atherosclerosis develop?***

Since atherosclerosis is a change in the inner lining of the vessels, it generally arises from changes in the composition and flow properties of the blood. Elevated blood lipids lead to the formation of fatty plaques. Elevated **blood pressure values** as well as **turbulence** within the vessel lead to deposits of **calcium** and **hardening** of the vessel wall. This also creates irregularities, so the vessel wall is no longer as smooth as before. This in turn attracts **platelets** (thrombocytes), which additionally adhere to the calcium deposits. This accelerates the formation of deposits and the narrowing increases (see Fig. 2).

11. ***Are there vessels that are more frequently affected?***

In principle, all arteries in the body, from head to toe, can be affected by atherosclerosis. However, there are vessels that are more frequently affected or in which involvement can lead to serious problems. Table 1 provides an overview.

12. ***What diseases can result from atherosclerosis?***

Since atherosclerosis can affect all the arteries throughout the body, the resulting diseases are very diverse. Ultimately, both pathological narrowings (stenoses) and the opposite, namely dilations (aneurysms), can occur. Narrowings arise from the deposits of fats, cholesterol, and calcium. Dilations result from the altered resilience of the vessel wall, which can lead to bulging and even rupture.

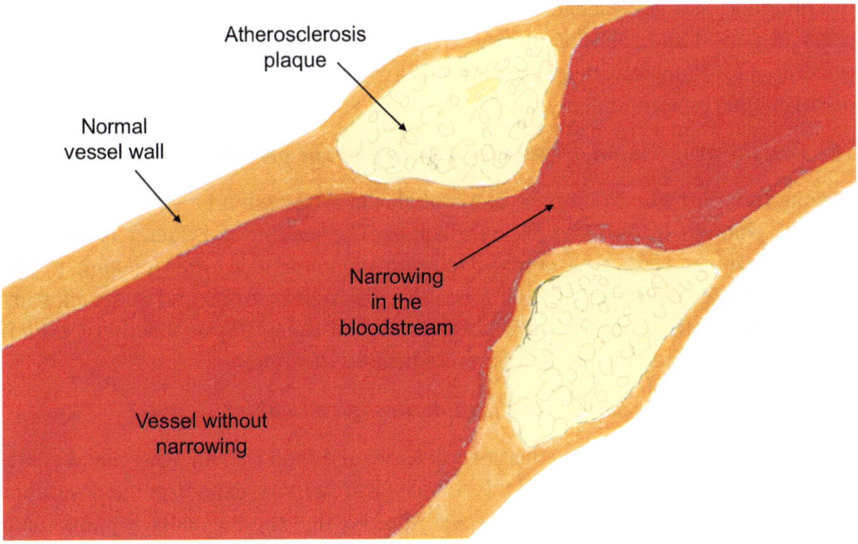

Fig. 2 Schematic representation of atherosclerotic plaques in an artery

Table 1 Overview of arteries frequently affected by atherosclerosis and resulting diseases

Affected vessel	Disease	Relevant specialty
Carotid arteries	Stroke	Vascular surgery
Coronary arteries	Heart attack	Cardiac surgery/Cardiology
Abdominal aorta	Ruptured aneurysm	Vascular surgery
Thoracic aorta	Ruptured aneurysm	Vascular surgery
Mesenteric artery	Bowel infarction ("black bowel")	Vascular surgery
Femoral/leg artery	Arterial occlusion ("cold leg")	Vascular surgery

13. ***What examinations can be used to detect atherosclerosis?***

The simplest and fastest examination is ultrasound. This allows assessment of the vessel wall as well as the vessel lumen. Ultrasound (also referred to medically as sonography) has no side effects, can be repeated as often as needed, and enables the examiner to detect calcifications and narrowings, as well as bulges and deposits in the vessel wall. In addition, vascular occlusions can be visualized, as blood flow is no longer detectable in these areas.

14. ***Are there medications that can dissolve calcifications?***

Once calcifications have formed, they are firmly attached to the arterial wall and cannot be dissolved by medication. Flat fatty deposits, which are already observed in childhood and adolescence, can regress. However, if these deposits persist for a longer period and calcifications have developed, simple dissolution is no longer possible. Unfortunately, there are currently (still) no medications available that can dissolve atherosclerotic deposits.

15. ***Can the progression of vascular calcification be prevented?***

Among the most important measures to halt the progression of vascular calcification are changes in diet and lifestyle habits. The leading risk factor is smoking, which is why it cannot be emphasized and recommended often enough to quit smoking. Other measures include a healthy diet rich in fruits and vegetables and low in industrially processed foods high in fat and sugar. Physical activity, even in the form of simple walks, is also part of a healthy lifestyle.

16. ***Can I prevent vascular calcification through a healthy lifestyle?***

Since atherosclerosis is a degenerative disease, and thus also an age-related condition, even a healthy diet and plenty of physical activity cannot prevent vascular calcifications from developing. However, the risk that these usually asymptomatic (= not causing any problems) vascular calcifications will lead to complications can be significantly reduced by a health-conscious lifestyle. For example, it is entirely normal for a 75-year-old woman who is very healthy and leads a healthy lifestyle to have occasional calcified deposits in her vessels. This in itself is not pathological, but rather a completely normal sign of aging.

Intermittent Claudication (Literally: "shop Window Disease")

17. ***What exactly is peripheral artery disease (PAD)?***

Peripheral artery disease (medically: claudicatio intermittens) refers to the narrowing of the arteries in the legs, which in the vast majority of cases is caused by atherosclerosis. Due to this arterial narrowing, the blood flow to the leg muscles can no longer be increased and maintained during exertion. This means that leg pain occurs during physical activity, which disappears completely at rest. Therefore, a typical feature of PAD is that patients repeatedly take breaks while walking to reduce the strain on their legs and relieve the pain. After these rest periods, patients are once again able to tolerate temporary exertion.

18. ***How and why does peripheral artery disease develop?***

Peripheral artery disease develops when the arteries (medically: arteries) in the legs develop narrowings or blockages, caused by deposits of calcium, fats, and cholesterol crystals in the vessel wall. As we age, the vessel wall naturally becomes less elastic, which increases the risk of deposits and narrowing. In principle, all arteries can be affected in PAD—from the large abdominal aorta (aorta) to the pelvic arteries (iliac arteries), the groin, and down to the arteries of the thigh and lower leg. However, the groin and thigh vessels are most commonly affected. The femoral arteries in the groin are usually narrowed and are easily accessible for surgery. In the thigh, narrowings above the knee joint or long-segment occlusions are often observed.

19. ***How high is the risk of developing peripheral artery disease?***

This cannot be answered in general terms and depends on how old you are or will become. The risk of developing PAD increases with age. It is estimated that one in four people over the age of 75 is affected, and by age 80, one in three.

In Germany, there is also a rising trend in the number of people affected. In 2000, just over 1% of the population (about 1 million) was affected; 20 years later,

S. Regus, *Answering Patients' Questions About Vascular Medicine*,
https://doi.org/10.1007/978-3-662-72771-3_3

the figure was nearly 3% (2.5 million???). This increase is attributed, among other things, to rising life expectancy, but also to our lifestyle and dietary habits.[1]

Everyone can do something to reduce their risk, but there is no guaranteed way to prevent peripheral artery disease.

20. ***Can I prevent peripheral artery disease through healthy eating and regular exercise?***

Peripheral artery disease is primarily caused by atherosclerosis, with deposits of calcium and cholesterol in the vessel wall. These deposits naturally develop over the course of life and become increasingly common with age. From this perspective, PAD is an age-related condition over which aging individuals generally have little or no control. Dying young would be an option, but not a good one: we all wish for a long and healthy life. The good news, however, is that everyone can influence the extent of vascular calcification. Regular physical activity, a varied and healthy diet, and avoiding overweight and nicotine can significantly delay the onset and reduce the severity of vascular calcification.

So the answer to the question is that everyone can make a significant contribution to reducing their risk of vascular calcification.

21. ***Do I have to be afraid of losing my leg if I have peripheral artery disease?***

In principle, every vascular disease carries risks, including advanced circulatory disorders, infection, and, in extreme cases, loss of the limb. However, in PAD, there is usually a compensated circulatory disorder, meaning the body has developed collateral circulation to compensate, so the risk of amputation is low. Nevertheless, you should watch for signs of worsening circulation. These include nighttime resting pain that improves when the leg is dangled out of bed (see Fig. 1).

But open wounds that heal poorly should also prompt you to seek medical attention.

22. ***Can I develop a sudden arterial blockage if I have peripheral artery disease?***

Normally, in peripheral artery disease, symptoms of poor circulation only occur when the leg is under strain. A sudden arterial blockage (medically: acute arterial occlusion) usually causes very severe pain and a cold sensation in the leg. These symptoms are independent of activity and therefore also occur at rest. This distinguishes a sudden arterial blockage from PAD. However, it can happen that clots

---

[1] Rammos C, Steinmetz M, Lortz J, Mahabadi AA, Petrikhovich O, Kirsch K, Hering R, Schulz M, Rassaf T. Peripheral artery disease in Germany (2009–2018): Prevalence, frequency of specialized ambulatory care and use of guideline-recommended therapy – A population-based study. Lancet Reg Health Eur. 2021 May 3;5:100113. doi: https://doi.org/10.1016/j.lanepe.2021.100113. PMID: 34557822; PMCID: PMC8454876.

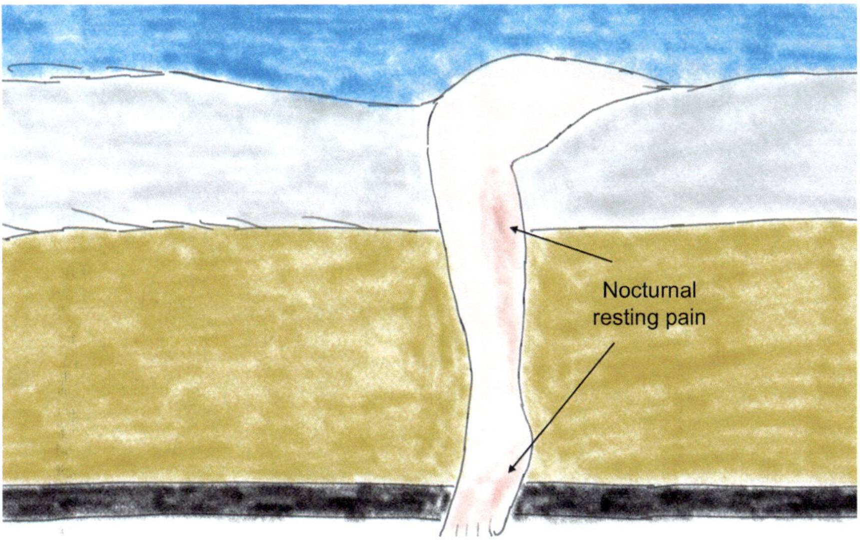

Fig. 1 With nighttime resting pain, the leg is typically dangled out of bed to improve blood flow and relieve symptoms

form in the narrowed vessels in PAD, which can then lead to a sudden arterial blockage. For this reason, many patients with PAD are advised to take blood thinners. This can significantly reduce the risk of clot formation. Typically, acetylsalicylic acid, also known as ASA® or Godamed®, is prescribed. Therefore, you should not discontinue these blood thinners on your own without first consulting your doctor. Strictly speaking, these are not "blood thinners" (an example of which would be Marcumar®), but rather medications that inhibit the clumping of platelets (thrombocytes) and thus reduce clot formation. They are also known as platelet aggregation inhibitors.

23. ***Is such an occlusion of the femoral artery not very painful and dangerous?***

The occlusion of the femoral artery is, in itself, neither painful nor dangerous. This is because the occlusion usually develops over many months and years, progressing from increasing narrowing to complete blockage. As a result, collateral circulation typically develops, which is often as effective as the main artery (see Fig. 2). You can imagine it similarly to a highway and the surrounding country roads: if one or more lanes on the highway are closed, the country roads are used. The body can also reinforce and expand its "country roads," so that, in the end, it may even be faster to travel via the "country roads" than the "highway." This is also the main principle behind walking training.

24. ***Are there different forms of peripheral artery disease (PAD)?***

Ultimately, there are different degrees of severity in peripheral artery disease. The severity can usually be assessed based on the walking distance, which is why,

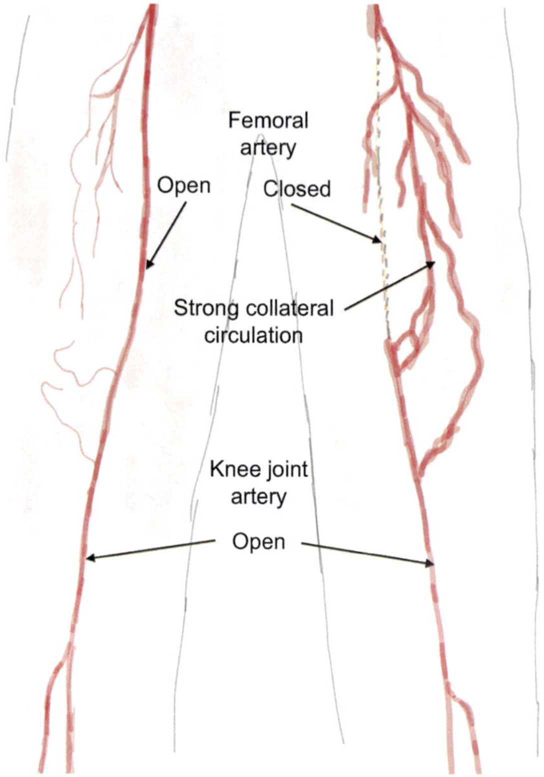

Fig. 2 Schematic representation of collateralization (development of bypass circuits) in an occlusion of the femoral artery

during a vascular surgical examination, the pain-free walking distance is always inquired about. Ideally, this should be specified in meters; if not possible, a so-called "walking distance test" can be performed on a treadmill. It is also crucial to determine whether and to what extent the patient feels their quality of life is impaired. For example, a person of very advanced age may be perfectly content and able to manage daily life with just 20 meters of walking within their home, whereas a younger, more active patient may find a pain-free walking distance of 500 meters insufficient. Consider, for instance, a mail carrier.

25. ***What examinations are performed for peripheral artery disease?***

The most important step in clarifying peripheral artery disease is certainly taking the **medical history**, which is also referred to medically as the **anamnesis**. Here, risk factors for vascular calcification are assessed, particularly the presence of poorly controlled high blood pressure or diabetes mellitus, high blood lipids, and smoking.

Also important in this context is obtaining a **family history**, especially whether vascular diseases (such as stroke or heart attack) are common in the family or have occurred, and whether they may have been the cause of death in a close relative.

The next important examination for suspected peripheral artery disease is the **measurement of blood pressure at the foot**, with particular emphasis on comparison with the blood pressure at the arm. The technical term for this examination is the ankle-brachial Doppler index, often abbreviated as **ABI** (from the English **A**nkle **B**rachial **I**ndex). Normally, the blood pressure at the foot is as high as at the arm. If the blood pressure at the foot is lower than at the arm, this, above a certain threshold, also indicates a circulatory disorder and should be further investigated.

In such cases, an ultrasound examination (sonography) can be performed, which often provides more precise information about changes and calcification in the vessel walls, as well as about narrowings or occlusions of arteries.

For further therapy planning and selection of the appropriate treatment method, an MR angiography is often subsequently ordered. This is also referred to as **MR (magnetic resonance) angiography** and is simply abbreviated as **MRA**.

26. ***Are stents the only treatment option for peripheral artery disease?***

The use of stents is certainly one of the most important and now also most frequently used options for treating early-stage peripheral artery disease. However, there are a variety of other treatment methods, for example:

- Walking training
- Medications to improve blood flow
- Removal of calcified deposits via catheter
- Surgical removal of calcified plaques, including suturing in of patch grafts
- Bypassing vascular occlusions with a bypass graft

27. ***What is the principle of walking training?***

Walking training involves structured exertion of the leg muscles and their blood supply through regular walking, continuing until pain occurs. Then, short breaks are taken, and walking resumes until the burning pain in the calves or thighs returns. Strictly speaking, it is comparable to muscle training in a gym. In walking training, the specific leg muscles are exercised through regular sessions, by alternating walking with rest and repeating this cycle several times. This training increases blood flow to the muscles, and collateral circulation—essentially new blood vessels—develops. These new vessels, also called collateral vessels, can bypass narrowings and occlusions in the original arteries. You can imagine it like a highway closure and subsequent traffic diversion onto country roads. Although these "side routes" are usually slower, if there are enough of them, you can still reach your destination without traffic jams.

28. ***What medications can be taken for peripheral artery disease?***

The most commonly prescribed medication for vascular calcification, and thus also for peripheral artery disease, is **acetylsalicylic acid**. This medication is also known as ASA® or Godamed®. It prevents blood platelets from adhering to calcified areas of the vessel wall, thereby reducing the risk of sudden vascular occlusions or worsening of narrowings.

Another medication is cilostazol, known by the trade name Pletal®. This drug, in combination with walking training, leads to a more rapid increase in pain-free walking distance.

So-called **cholesterol-lowering agents**, known as **statins**, are also frequently prescribed. They are also prescribed even when blood values and, in particular, cholesterol are within the normal range, which often surprises patients. The purpose of **statins** (for example, simvastatin, atorvastatin) in these cases is less to lower blood lipids and more to stabilize calcified deposits. Studies have shown that statin therapy makes calcified deposits in the vessels less fissured and slows their growth. In peripheral artery disease, this primarily affects the leg vessels, but statins also slow the progression of calcified deposits and smooth the surface of plaques in all other vessels.

Some patients are also recommended a **stronger blood thinning** therapy, which is administered in the hospital via injections and infusions, and outside the hospital usually in the form of tablets.

These stronger blood-thinning medications include the so-called **Marcumar®** (active ingredient phenprocoumon), which is prescribed especially after complicated bypass procedures. Marcumar® is also frequently recommended for cardiac arrhythmias. The disadvantage of Marcumar® is that regular laboratory monitoring is necessary to determine and adjust the correct dosage. Experience shows that this can range from 1/4 tablet every other day to 2 tablets daily.

There are now newer medications that can be dosed the same for all patients, making regular blood tests unnecessary. These medications are collectively referred to as "**n**ew **o**ral **an**ticoagulants (NOACs)." **Oral** means that the medication is taken by mouth in tablet form. **Anti** stands for "against," and **coagulation** is the technical term for clotting. Examples of NOACs include **Xarelto®** (active ingredient rivaroxaban) or **Eliquis®** (active ingredient apixaban). However, these blood-thinning medications can at best reduce the symptoms of peripheral artery disease and slow the progression of the disease. They cannot dissolve calcified deposits or eliminate narrowings or vascular occlusions. For this, a balloon dilation or vascular surgery is required.

29. ***What surgical procedures are available?***

For short narrowings and occlusions, it is possible to open the vessel at the narrowed site and remove the deposits. However, the vessel cannot be closed directly afterward, as this would result in an hourglass-shaped narrowing at that site. Instead, it is necessary to suture in a patch, a procedure known as patch angioplasty.

For long-segment narrowings or occlusions, which can sometimes be 20 cm or longer, patch angioplasty is complex and less promising. In such cases, a so-called **bypass** is created. This is a detour that bridges the blocked vessel. Often, the patient's own vein from the leg is used for this purpose, but sometimes synthetic

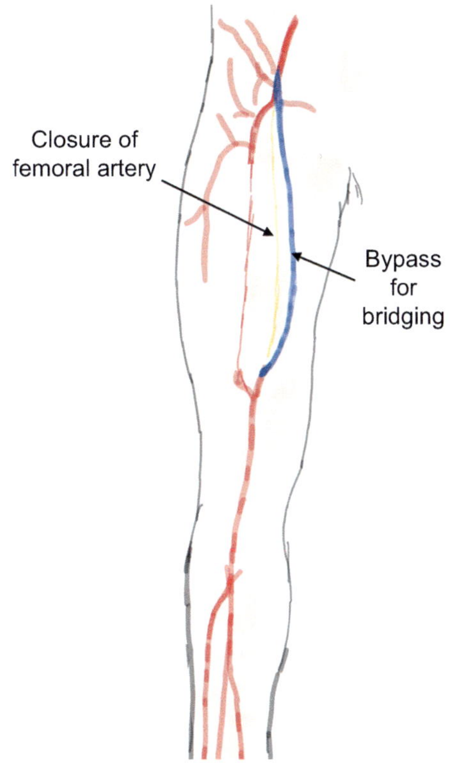

Fig. 3 Schematic representation of a bypass in the leg to bridge a vascular occlusion

material (plastic) must be used. Most people associate the word bypass with heart surgery. While this is not incorrect—bypasses can also be performed on the heart—this becomes necessary when the coronary arteries are blocked or narrowed and a stent cannot be placed or has repeatedly become blocked. Heart bypasses are performed by cardiac surgeons. However, a bypass can also be necessary in all other vessels, such as in the leg or the main abdominal artery (see Fig. 3).

The most common reason for this is peripheral artery disease. Bypass surgery is a very common standard vascular surgical therapy.

Chronic Wounds

30. ***What do wounds have to do with blood circulation?***

Every skin injury requires effective wound healing in order to close up and form a healthy skin surface again. Wound healing involves supplying the wound with nutrients and oxygen, as well as removing foreign bodies, bacteria, and tissue breakdown products. All of this depends on a healthy and functional vascular system, which is why the vascular system should always be evaluated in cases of chronic wounds or delayed wound healing.

31. ***When is a wound considered chronic?***

If a wound does not heal over a longer period, this is referred to in medicine as a wound healing disorder or chronic wound. Usually, a period of 8 weeks is considered the threshold at which an acute (fresh) wound becomes a poorly healing (chronic) wound. However, there are underlying conditions in which every wound is considered chronic from the outset. This includes, for example, diabetes mellitus, as patients with this condition have impaired wound healing from the start. This is mainly because elevated blood sugar levels delay the natural wound healing process.

32. ***How many people have chronic wounds?***

In Germany, about 2–4 million people suffer from a chronic wound. This means that about 2–5 out of every 100 patients are affected. Chronic wounds are therefore among the most common diseases and are often a reason for hospitalization. Increasingly, however, chronic wounds are also being treated on an outpatient basis, which is why wound care and specially trained wound managers are becoming ever more important.

S. Regus, *Answering Patients' Questions About Vascular Medicine*,
https://doi.org/10.1007/978-3-662-72771-3_4

33. ***What are the most common causes of chronic, non-healing wounds?***

By far the most common cause is diabetes mellitus, which is referred to as a lifestyle disease in highly developed countries. This condition is often associated with lack of physical activity and obesity, both of which are significant risk factors for the development of wounds. This is evident from the fact that almost half of people with obesity and lack of exercise suffer from a chronic wound at least once in their lives. However, vascular diseases, especially circulatory disorders such as peripheral arterial occlusive disease (PAOD) or chronic venous insufficiency, are also important causes.

34. ***Which clinical pictures are characterized by chronic wounds?***

There are a variety of diseases associated with chronic wounds and wound healing disorders. In PAOD, as a circulatory disorder, non-healing wounds often develop on the toes as well as around the lateral malleolus or the outer side of the lower leg.

Venous diseases can also lead to chronic wounds, which, however, are typically located around the inner ankle. They can also extend circumferentially, i.e., around the entire lower leg.

Diabetes mellitus, the most common metabolic disease in our affluent society, often leads to wounds and inflammation of the toes. In gout, inflammation and pain typically occur in the big toe. Skin diseases can also frequently result in poorly healing wounds that require further investigation.

It is therefore generally advisable to seek medical examination and clarification in cases of poor wound healing.

35. ***What examinations are necessary for chronic wounds?***

Several examinations are indicated for chronic wounds. Most often, the vascular supply needs to be assessed, which is done using special blood pressure measurements on the foot and an ultrasound examination. In addition, it may be necessary to examine the wound for bacteria and other pathogens. This is usually done by taking wound swabs and examining them under a microscope. Blood or urine tests are also often required to clarify metabolic diseases in the context of chronic wounds.

36. ***How are chronic wounds treated?***

Ultimately, two aspects are important in the treatment of chronic wounds: First and foremost is, of course, the treatment of the wound surface with special wound dressings and bandages. This promotes healing of the wound surface. In addition, treating the underlying disease, such as diabetes mellitus or PAOD, is also important to create the best possible conditions for undisturbed wound healing.

37. ***Do I have to stay in the hospital until my wounds are healed?***

In the vast majority of cases, it is not necessary for patients with chronic wounds to remain in the hospital until the wound has healed (which can take several weeks or months). Rather, an initial surgical wound cleaning and regular dressing changes (initially daily, then every 2–3 days) are performed. Once the wound conditions are stable—meaning wound healing has been activated and the wound is clean and able to heal—further wound care can be provided on an outpatient basis. For this, a dressing service is often organized, for example by a nursing service or a wound manager.

38. ***What are my chances that my chronic wound will heal?***

This question cannot be answered in general terms, as the healing process and duration depend very much on the causes, the nature, and the size of the wound. Uncomplicated wound healing usually takes about 2 weeks, which is also the typical time for a surgical wound to heal. Large wound areas, poor circulation, or infections, on the other hand, delay wound healing, which can then take several months.

39. ***What can I do myself to prevent my wounds from becoming chronic?***

If there are no other conditions that impair wound healing (such as diabetes mellitus, gout, or rheumatism), good skin care and protective dressings are usually sufficient. Chronic wounds typically only develop in the presence of additional vascular diseases (arteries or veins) or in the context of metabolic or immune system disorders. In some cases, impaired wound healing may indicate an as yet undiagnosed underlying disease.

Amputations

40. ***What does "amputate" actually mean?***

To amputate means to remove a part of the body. The term comes from Latin ("amputare" meaning to take off, cut off, shorten) and is used in medicine whenever significant portions of tissue and organs are completely removed. For example, the removal of the rectum along with the sphincter muscle is referred to as a rectal amputation. Most commonly, however, the term amputation is used in connection with the removal of extremities, such as an arm or leg. In these cases, the part of the extremity that is removed is specified, for example, toe, lower leg, or thigh amputation.

41. ***What is meant by "salami tactics"?***

"Salami tactics" refers to performing an amputation in several stages. The background is that doctors (usually at the explicit request of the patient) try to remove as little diseased tissue as possible and preserve as much as they can. This is often the case with "black toes." Here, in the hope that the wound will heal, only the diseased and dead toe is initially removed. However, if blood circulation is insufficient or the infection is too advanced, it often happens that the wound does not heal and the amputation must be continued at a higher level. Even then, it can happen that the wound still does not heal and another higher-level amputation is necessary. Although the term "salami tactics" has a negative reputation, the intention behind it is the good faith effort of physicians to preserve as much healthy tissue as possible. Alternatively, if wound healing is predictably unlikely, the amputation should be performed at the level where healing can be expected. This approach prevents "salami tactics," but many patients and their relatives are initially shocked by the information that the entire lower leg or even part of the knee must be removed.

S. Regus, *Answering Patients' Questions About Vascular Medicine*,
https://doi.org/10.1007/978-3-662-72771-3_5

42. ***When does the foot need to be amputated?***

The decisive factor for the level of amputation above the ankle joint, including removal of the entire foot, is the extent of tissue damage. It is also crucial whether the foot can be preserved and remains functional. For example, a large wound (medically: ulceration) in the area of the heel and sole can result in the foot being permanently unable to bear weight. In such cases, amputation of the entire foot may be preferable to enable the patient to regain mobility with a prosthesis. Accidents can also cause such severe damage to the foot or ankle joint that amputation becomes unavoidable. Ultimately, advanced infection of the ankle joint, leading to pus accumulation in the joint cavity, is also a reason for amputation of the entire foot including the ankle. In cases of circulatory disorders, it is necessary, if required, to first attempt improvement with balloon dilation, stent placement, or a bypass procedure.

43. ***Why does my leg have to be removed above the knee joint?***

In principle, the goal is to remove as little diseased tissue as possible, but as much as necessary. Therefore, amputation above the knee joint is only necessary when there is extensive soft tissue damage, advanced infection, or significant circulatory disorder. For example, a severe accident can cause such massive soft tissue damage that only an amputation above the knee joint offers a chance of healing. Likewise, infection of the entire foot, including pus accumulation in the ankle and knee joints, can constitute a so-called indication for amputation. Ultimately, advanced vascular occlusions or multiple previous bypass procedures in the leg with recurrent blockages may also necessitate amputation above the knee to save the patient's life. In such cases, the principle applies: "Life before limb" (meaning: "Life comes first and is more important than the leg").

44. ***Why do diabetics have a higher risk of amputation?***

Statistically, diabetics have a higher risk of amputation than non-diabetics. This means that diabetics are more likely to undergo limb amputation, and the proportion of diabetics among patients who undergo amputation is higher than that of non-diabetics. However, this does not mean that diabetics inherently have a high risk of amputation or are highly likely to lose a leg during their lifetime. The particular aspect of diabetes in relation to amputation risk is that, firstly, wound healing is significantly delayed, and secondly, open wounds and pressure points on the foot are often noticed too late or not at all by the patient. This is due to so-called diabetic polyneuropathy, a disease of the nerves. This nerve disorder leads to reduced pain sensitivity. The combination of diabetic angiopathy (vascular disease) and polyneuropathy (nerve disease) is the reason for the increased risk of amputation in diabetics.

45. *Why did I first receive a bypass and now my leg still has to be amputated?*

When there is advanced circulatory disorder, it may be necessary to place a bypass in the leg. Ideally, this will allow the damaged tissue to recover and avoid the need for amputation. However, it can also happen that the limb (the leg) does not recover despite the bypass, and surgery is still required. This may also be necessary if there is an infection or pus accumulations develop. In particularly severe cases, the principle always applies: Life before limb!

At the latest, when large tissue defects or blood poisoning threaten life, amputation is indicated.

46. *Can I walk with a leg prosthesis?*

After a toe amputation, a leg prosthesis is usually not necessary to enable walking. However, special footwear may be required to relieve pressure on the fresh surgical wound and to allow for wearing a dressing inside the shoe.

The situation is different after an amputation above the ankle joint or including the knee joint. In these cases, a prosthesis is generally necessary to enable mobility. Depending on the level of activity before the amputation, special prostheses can even allow for sports, including competitive sports (keyword: Paralympics). Therefore, physical therapy is strongly recommended if a prosthesis is planned. In some cases, however, a prosthesis is not pursued from the outset if the patient was already unable to walk before the amputation and is very frail. If, however, there is significant improvement in the patient's condition in the weeks or months following the amputation, a prosthesis can still be considered.

47. *Do I have to go to rehab after the amputation?*

If patients are fit and were able to walk well before the amputation, every effort should be made to fit a prosthesis. With this leg prosthesis, many patients can lead a normal life and remain active. However, this requires a well-fitting prosthesis and active practice and training. All of this takes place as part of a rehabilitation program, often directly following the hospital stay. In a so-called rehabilitation clinic, walking with the prosthesis is practiced under the guidance of a physical therapist, and muscle strengthening is performed. Treatment there usually lasts 3–4 weeks and can also be done on an outpatient basis. However, for prosthesis training, inpatient care is usually better suited to help patients regain mobility more quickly and achieve targeted muscle strengthening.

48. *Why do some people still feel their foot after a leg amputation?*

After an amputation, so-called phantom pain can occur, in which the patient still feels the removed limb. For example, the patient may report pain in the foot, even though it is no longer present. Phantom pain arises because nerve endings at the level of the amputation are severed but can still be activated. This creates the illusion in the brain that the foot is still there and experiencing pain.

49. ***How many people in Germany wear a leg prosthesis after amputation?***

The number of people in Germany who rely on a leg prosthesis is very small, at around 150,000. That is only about 2‰ of the population, or 2 out of every 1000 inhabitants. Most leg prosthesis users are over 65 years old and have lost their leg due to circulatory disorders. Young people rarely require a leg prosthesis, and in the majority of cases, they have undergone amputation as a result of an accident or a tumor. However, younger people are much more likely and able to walk again with a leg prosthesis and manage their daily lives, even participate in sports. For older people, this is often much more difficult due to accompanying frailty, reduced muscle mass, and pre-existing limited mobility. Many seniors remain only in their homes, whereas younger patients were usually very mobile and physically active before the accident.

50. ***How great is the risk that an amputation will become necessary?***

Fortunately, the risk that amputation of a limb (especially the leg) will become necessary is very low. In Germany, about 60,000 amputations are performed each year. With a population of 80 million, this affects 1‰ of the population, or one in a thousand. In the majority of cases, these are so-called minor amputations, which include all "small amputations," especially toe amputations. A major amputation, on the other hand, means that at least the foot or even the knee joint must be removed. In numbers: per 100,000 inhabitants, about 60 amputations are necessary each year, of which 45 are minor amputations. Major amputations account for about 15 per 100,000 inhabitants. More than 50% of lower and upper leg amputations ("major") affect diabetics, which again highlights the significance of diabetes as a risk factor for amputation. It cannot be emphasized enough that good blood sugar control in diabetics and the consistent avoidance of pressure points from ill-fitting footwear are essential for preventing amputation.

51. ***Why do diabetics have a comparatively high risk of losing their leg?***

The particularity in diabetics is that, in addition to circulatory disorders, they also have nerve damage and increased susceptibility to infections. Due to their circulatory disorders and vascular calcifications, they experience poorer wound healing, which is also the case in patients with peripheral arterial occlusive disease (PAOD).

In diabetics, there are also vascular changes in nerves, especially sensory nerves, which are responsible for pressure and pain sensitivity. This leads to diabetics being less able to feel pressure points and wounds on the foot, resulting in the loss of the natural protective mechanism. This means that, in diabetics, wounds develop more quickly due to unrecognized pressure points and, because of continued pressure, do not heal properly. In addition, diabetics have an increased risk of infection, meaning that infections on the foot develop more quickly and can spread and worsen rapidly. One reason for this is their reduced immune defense.

52. ***Which diseases put you at risk of losing your leg?***

There are various causes that can lead to the loss of a leg. The most common cause among older people in our society is circulatory disorder (PAOD). This common disease is also known as "window shopper's disease." Another disease that can lead to leg amputation is diabetes mellitus, commonly referred to as diabetes. In diabetes mellitus, circulatory disorder is also the main issue, but there is also a risk of developing severe infections. Accidents are the most common cause of amputations in younger people, but fortunately, they are very rare. The same applies to malignant tumors, which can force the removal of a leg in childhood. This is also very rare, but in individual cases, it can have very serious consequences for the child.

53. ***What types of amputations are there?***

In principle, amputations are classified according to which limb is involved. The main distinction is whether it is the upper limb (arm and hand) or the lower limb (leg and foot). The next important factor is the level at which the limb is amputated. Since lower limb amputation is by far the most common, it is further classified (from bottom to top) into toe, foot, lower leg, and thigh amputation. Amputation at or including the hip joint is fortunately very rare. It is also important to distinguish between open and closed amputation. In a closed amputation, the skin is sutured; in an open amputation, the skin is not sutured. The latter may be necessary if an infection is present and closing the skin would perpetuate the infection.

54. ***Why does the leg sometimes have to be removed above the knee joint?***

In severe cases of circulatory disorder or very advanced tissue damage, it may be necessary to remove the entire leg, including the knee joint. Whenever possible, however, every effort should be made to preserve the knee joint, as the patient will be able to sit or transfer (for example, from bed to wheelchair) more easily even without a prosthesis. Fitting a leg prosthesis is also much easier if the knee joint is preserved. In cases of severe injuries after accidents or severe soft tissue infections that extend beyond the knee to the thigh, amputation including the knee joint often becomes unavoidable. This should be explained in detail to the patient and their relatives so that this difficult decision can be made. Exceptions are emergency situations after serious traffic accidents, in which the patient's life would be at risk without amputation. In these cases, the principle applies: Life before limb ("Life is more important than the leg").

55. ***When is it sufficient to amputate only a toe or parts of the foot?***

In some cases, it may be sufficient to remove only the affected toe. This is possible, for example, in the case of an isolated "black toe." However, it is important to rule out or treat a circulatory disorder of the leg before amputation. Therefore, before any amputation, even a "minor toe amputation," an examination of the arteries is absolutely necessary in order to perform angioplasty or a bypass if needed. Otherwise, there is a risk that the surgical wound will not heal and further procedures will be required. In exceptional situations, the toe is amputated immediately and the vascular examination is performed afterward. This is always the case when the toe is infected with pus and blood poisoning is present or imminent. In such cases, the toe must be removed as an emergency to prevent infection or sepsis.

56. ***How great is the risk that I will also lose the other leg?***

This question cannot be answered in general terms, as the answer depends in particular on the cause and the reasons that necessitated the amputation. After a so-called traumatic leg amputation, which is due to an accident and severe injury, the risk of amputation of the opposite leg is very low. Of course, this assumes that the opposite leg was not also injured during the accident. The situation is different for amputations that had to be performed due to peripheral arterial occlusive disease or diabetes mellitus. Both of these are so-called systemic diseases, which are not limited to one leg but affect the entire body. Therefore, in these cases, the risk to the opposite leg is also increased and, in poorly controlled diabetes mellitus, can be as high as 30%. This makes consistent wound care and the treatment of diabetes mellitus all the more important to avoid complications such as amputation.

57. ***Do I have to expect that the "salami tactic" will be used on me?***

The approach commonly referred to as the "salami tactic" in amputations means that a leg is removed slice by slice. For example, first a toe is removed, then several toes, eventually the foot and lower leg, up to the thigh. This may become necessary if, on the one hand, an attempt is made to remove as little tissue as possible, but on the other hand, the blood supply is insufficient to achieve wound healing. In such cases, repeated surgeries are required to finally achieve healing of the amputation wound. It is often possible to anticipate in advance that an amputation will not heal. Then, through careful planning of the amputation level (i.e., whether toe, foot, lower leg, or thigh is sufficient), the salami tactic and thus multiple surgical interventions can be avoided. However, many patients are alarmed when they are initially recommended an above-knee amputation. In these cases, thorough patient education and an explanation of the circumstances as to why an amputation of the toes or just the foot should be avoided are essential and important for the healing process.

58. ***How can amputations be prevented?***

The most important measures to prevent amputations in diabetics are the consistent and good control of blood glucose levels and the avoidance of foot wounds caused by pressure points. In patients with PAD and the resulting circulatory disorders of the leg, however, it is necessary to eliminate vascular stenoses or even occlusions. In some cases, balloon dilation is sufficient (Fig. 1), but sometimes a bypass is necessary (Fig. 2).

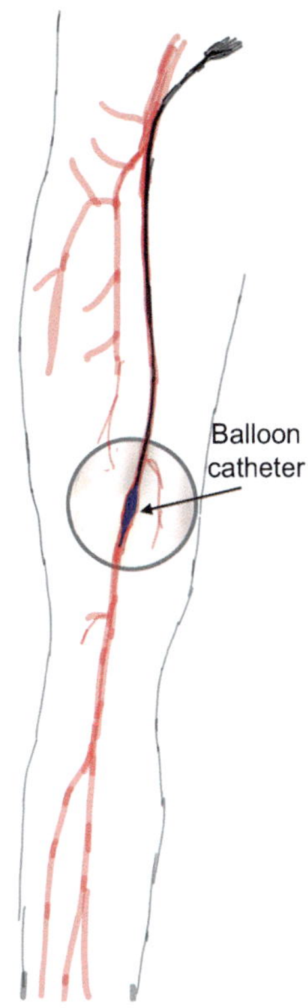

Fig. 1 A narrowing of the popliteal artery is dilated using a balloon

After accidents and extensive injuries to a leg, especially in the case of vascular injuries, rapid surgical intervention and restoration of blood flow can reduce the risk of amputation.

In the case of an extensive and serious condition, however, early indication for amputation is necessary, especially to avoid serious long-term consequences. Here, the already mentioned motto applies: "Life before limb."

Fig. 2 An occlusion of the femoral artery is bypassed with a graft

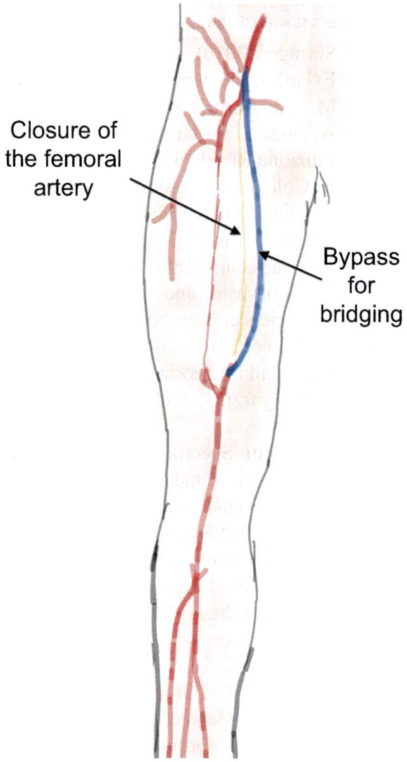

Diabetic Foot Syndrome

59. ***What exactly is the diabetic foot syndrome?***

The term "diabetic foot syndrome" encompasses all inflammations and chronic wounds of the foot that are caused by diabetes mellitus ("diabetes"). In principle, two mechanisms are primarily responsible for the development of diabetic foot syndrome. On the one hand, especially in long-standing diabetics, calcification of the vessel walls occurs, leading to circulatory disorders. On the other hand, diabetes mellitus also damages the nerves, resulting in reduced sensitivity in the foot. Thus, pressure points in the shoe, which are normally painful and would cause a person to remove the shoe, can lead to chronic pressure sores and wounds in diabetics with nerve damage (diabetic polyneuropathy). These wounds often become inflamed, which typically results in what is known as "diabetic foot syndrome."

60. ***How many diabetics have diabetic foot syndrome?***

About 6% of all diabetics currently have diabetic foot syndrome. The lifetime risk for a diabetic to develop diabetic foot syndrome is approximately 35%. This means that one in three diabetics will develop diabetic foot syndrome during their lifetime. Most cases of diabetic foot syndrome are temporary and heal, but in some cases, chronic, long-lasting open sores and wounds on the foot may develop. This should be avoided at all costs, as it not only significantly reduces quality of life but also greatly increases the risk of amputation.

61. ***Why should diabetics wear special shoes?***

Due to the nerve damage (diabetic polyneuropathy) that is often present in diabetics, pressure points can frequently develop on the foot and between the toes, but the diabetic hardly notices them. Because of the nerve damage, sensitivity in the foot is significantly reduced. As a result, pressure points can develop in regular shoes, quickly increase in size, and lead to ulceration. Such pressure points occur much less frequently in special shoes. Therefore, in addition to thorough foot care,

S. Regus, *Answering Patients' Questions About Vascular Medicine*,
https://doi.org/10.1007/978-3-662-72771-3_6

diabetics are advised to wear special offloading shoes. In most cases, these are custom adaptations that can be ordered from a medical supply store or specialized online retailers. There is now a wide variety of different models, many of which closely resemble regular shoes.

62. ***How great is the risk for a diabetic to develop diabetic foot syndrome?***

The likelihood that a diabetic will develop a poorly healing wound on the foot during their lifetime is high. It is estimated that every second diabetic is affected, although the patient's own self-care always plays a decisive role. Conscientious foot care can significantly reduce the risk. However, good blood sugar control is also of primary importance.

About one in three diabetics will develop diabetic foot syndrome during their lifetime, and here too, consistent self-care and foot care are the most important measures to prevent this.

63. ***Why does diabetic foot syndrome develop?***

The causes of diabetic foot syndrome are varied. The main factor is so-called diabetic angiopathy, i.e., circulatory disorders caused by calcification of the blood vessels. In diabetics, the small vessels that supply the foot and especially the toes are particularly affected. Another important cause is diabetic polyneuropathy, which refers to reduced pain sensitivity. This also develops as a result of diabetes mellitus, but in this case due to circulatory disorders of nerve tissue and the loss of nerve cells and fibers.

In addition to circulatory disorders, the blood sugar fluctuations that typically occur in diabetes mellitus are another cause of diabetic foot syndrome. This leads to nutritional disturbances in the tissue, which in turn result in impaired wound healing.

64. ***What different forms of diabetic foot syndrome are there?***

Diabetic foot syndrome is usually classified according to the extent of ulceration and whether there is an additional infection and/or circulatory disorder. The size and depth of the wound are described using the so-called Wagner grades (0–5), ranging from 0 (healed) through 1 (superficial) to 5 (deep, down to the bone). The accompanying factors are classified according to the Armstrong stages: A means that neither infection nor circulatory disorder is present, B means with infection, C with circulatory disorder, and D with both (i.e., with infection and circulatory disorder).

For the patient, this so-called Wagner-Armstrong classification has little consequence; for them, only the extent of the wound and the chance of healing are important. The classification is important for physicians to document and compare the course of the wound.

65. *What examinations can be used to diagnose diabetic foot syndrome?*

In the presence of diabetic foot syndrome with typical open wounds and foot deformities, a trained clinical eye is usually sufficient for diagnosis. Ideally, however, a patient at risk of developing diabetic foot syndrome is identified in advance. This can help prevent complications such as wounds, impaired wound healing, or even findings requiring amputation.

Examinations that can provide evidence of diabetic foot syndrome include, in particular, ultrasound of the arteries. In at-risk patients, this reveals narrowing of the vessels, especially in the lower leg or foot. An X-ray examination of the foot and lower leg can also provide initial indications of diabetic foot syndrome, but changes on X-ray usually indicate an advanced stage. An MRI scan can also provide important information and is often ordered in advanced stages. This can show changes in the bone as well as in joint and soft tissue structures.

With the tuning fork test, changes in nerve function, i.e., diabetic neuropathy, can be detected. For this, a vibrating tuning fork is placed on the foot and ankle, and it is assessed how long the increasingly weaker vibrations are perceived. If there are limitations compared to a healthy foot, this indicates diabetic neuropathy.

66. *Does every case of diabetic foot syndrome require amputation?*

Even though diabetic foot syndrome is a serious condition, it by no means always requires amputation. On the contrary: ideally, before complications arise, wound cleaning and regular dressing changes can achieve healing of the wounds. In addition, wearing appropriate offloading shoes and using special dressing materials can accelerate healing. Furthermore, to optimize blood flow, early dilation of vascular stenoses or placement of a bypass should be performed. For this reason, and to ensure nothing is overlooked, timely referral to vascular surgery is strongly recommended.

67. *How great is the risk that I will lose my leg if several toes have already been amputated?*

The risk of a so-called major amputation, that is, an amputation above the foot, is almost 50 times higher in diabetics compared to non-diabetics. At first, this sounds very alarming; however, considering the very low amputation rate in the general population, the number of amputations among diabetics is still to be regarded as rather low. According to the Federal Statistical Office, about 10 amputations per 100,000 diabetics are necessary each year. Male diabetics have a higher risk of amputation than female diabetics, although the reasons for this are not clearly understood. Diabetics who have previously undergone a toe amputation also have an increased risk of further amputation, but this does not mean that amputation hangs over the patient's head like the sword of Damocles. Every diabetic, whether or not they have had a previous toe amputation, has the opportunity to minimize their own risk of a major amputation.

68. ***What can I do myself to prevent an amputation?***

Regular visits to the doctor, good blood sugar control, and avoiding pressure points and wounds on the foot are important. Existing wounds should be regularly treated and monitored. Even if wearing special "diabetic shoes" may be uncomfortable, it should be done consistently. Only in this way can the worsening of wounds be prevented. This is particularly important because diabetics often feel wounds less, experience less pain, and therefore are less consistent in relieving pressure. In some cases, wearing special offloading orthoses may even be necessary. These are special shoes that extend up to the knee, provide support there, and thus completely relieve the foot. The foot is then virtually suspended in the shoe and bears no weight, allowing inflammation and wounds on the foot to heal better.

Vascular Occlusion

69. ***I have already had several thromboses in my leg; are these vascular occlusions?***

Strictly speaking, a thrombosis in the leg refers to clots that have formed in a deep vein of the leg. Causes for this include, for example, a long flight, surgery requiring immobilization of the leg, or blood clotting disorders. Swelling of the leg is the typical symptom of thromboses.

An acute vascular occlusion, on the other hand, refers to the sudden blockage of an artery. Here too, clots are often the cause, but the symptoms are completely different: there is no swelling of the leg, but rather a pronounced sensation of cold.

70. ***What causes an acute occlusion?***

An acute vascular occlusion can result from an arterial thrombosis or an embolism. In arterial thrombosis, a narrowing in the vessel forms a clot (also called a thrombus or thrombosis), which eventually causes a complete blockage. In contrast, an arterial embolism is a clot that forms not in the affected vessel but elsewhere, most often in the heart due to cardiac arrhythmias or in an outpouching of an artery, known as an aneurysm. This clot can then be carried by the bloodstream and become lodged in a vessel. In which artery the clot "gets stuck" depends primarily on its size. A large clot can, for example, cause a blockage in a pelvic artery, while a small clot can be carried as far as below the knee. It is important to note that in an embolism, the blocked vessel is generally healthy, whereas in thrombosis, the vessel is already diseased and narrowed beforehand. Consequently, risk factors and causes for an acute occlusion include a pre-existing narrowing due to atherosclerosis or an outpouching of arteries or cardiac arrhythmias.

S. Regus, *Answering Patients' Questions About Vascular Medicine*,
https://doi.org/10.1007/978-3-662-72771-3_7

71. ***Is a sudden vascular occlusion a common condition?***

A sudden vascular occlusion, medically referred to as acute vascular occlusion or, in clinical practice, as "cold leg" or "cold arm," is a relatively common condition treated in vascular surgery. Overall, it is a disease that primarily affects older patients who have cardiac arrhythmias or already suffer from atherosclerosis. The most common location for an acute occlusion is the leg, but the main aorta, the arm, and the brain (in the form of a stroke), as well as all abdominal vessels, can also be affected. Depending on the extent of the occlusion, it may be a condition that is easy to treat if only the arm or leg is involved, or an extremely complex situation if multiple vascular regions are affected.

72. ***Does a sudden vascular occlusion only occur in the leg?***

Arterial occlusion, also referred to as sudden vascular occlusion, can in principle occur in any artery. One of the most common locations is the leg, which is why patients often present to and are treated by vascular surgeons. However, in principle, any artery from head to toe can be affected. Since blood is pumped from the heart through the large thoracic and abdominal aorta directly into the legs, clots from the heart can be carried into the legs. These clots are the main cause of sudden vascular occlusion. Other locations include the brain or the arms, if the clot is diverted from the heart into the thoracic aorta and from there upwards (medically: cranially) and becomes lodged.

73. ***How can a vascular occlusion be detected and confirmed?***

A vascular occlusion can often be suspected based on the symptoms described by the patient. Typical symptoms are a sensation of cold, pain, and reduced sensitivity (numbness). In addition, the physical examination often raises suspicion of an acute vascular occlusion. Typically, one may find a foot that is cooler compared to the other side, reduced sensitivity to touch and pain, and a whitish or bluish discoloration. However, these are not definitive criteria; they only suggest an acute occlusion. More precise information is provided by ultrasound examination, while the best diagnostic confirmation can be obtained with a computed tomography (CT) or magnetic resonance imaging (MRI) scan.

74. ***Does a vascular occlusion always require surgery?***

There are several ways to treat a vascular occlusion. If the occlusion of an artery is due to a pre-existing narrowing, collateral circulation is often so well developed that the occlusion causes hardly any symptoms. In such cases, conservative therapy is recommended. This means that neither surgery nor catheter intervention is performed, but treatment is carried out solely with medication. This approach can avoid the side effects and complications of invasive therapy, such as surgery or balloon dilation. However, conservative management is only justified if the symptoms can be controlled with medication and there is no risk to the leg or the patient's life.

Catheter-based treatment is always possible when the narrowings or occlusions are relatively short and can be treated with balloons or stents.

Surgical intervention should be performed when there are long-segment occlusions and the circulatory problems are very pronounced. Surgical therapy, meaning exposure with skin incisions and removal of the clots as well as bypass grafting, is the fastest approach and is therefore usually indicated in cases of severe circulatory disorders. Only in this way can the leg be saved in cases of severe circulatory impairment. However, surgical procedures also carry risks, both for the leg and for all other vital organs such as the heart, lungs, and kidneys. Therefore, weighing all options and making the right decision in advance is extremely important.

75. ***Why do some people have to take a "blood thinner" after surgery and others do not?***

The majority of patients require blood thinning after a vascular occlusion. The type of blood thinning, however, depends on the type of vascular occlusion. If there is an embolic occlusion caused by a cardiac arrhythmia, a stronger blood thinner is necessary to prevent clot formation in the heart. These include, for example, Marcumar® (phenprocoumon) or one of the new blood thinners, such as Eliquis® (apixaban) or Xarelto® (rivaroxaban). The dosage of Marcumar, however, can only be determined by regular blood tests, which is not necessary with the so-called new blood thinners like Xarelto®. Here, a fixed dosage can be prescribed without daily blood tests, which is a major advantage.

If the cause of the arterial occlusion is vascular calcification (atherosclerosis), patients require a "lighter" blood thinner. In cases of vascular calcification, it is necessary to prevent clot formation by platelets and their deposition on the vessel wall. This is the mechanism of action of so-called antiplatelet agents such as aspirin (acetylsalicylic acid, ASS®) or Plavix® (clopidogrel).

If the vascular occlusion was caused by an accident, usually only temporary blood thinning is necessary; in cases of cardiac arrhythmias or vascular calcification, however, blood thinning is generally recommended and required for life.

76. ***What is the risk that the vascular occlusion will recur?***

This question cannot be answered in general terms. In the case of cardiac arrhythmias, it is crucial that anticoagulation is well and regularly managed and correctly dosed. The latter applies only to Marcumar®, whereas the new anticoagulants can be taken in a fixed dosage. With this, a renewed occlusion can most likely be prevented, but there is no absolute certainty. In atherosclerosis, it is decisive whether lifestyle changes are made, particularly whether sufficient physical activity and a healthy diet are observed. Smoking should also be stopped. Medications are also recommended for atherosclerosis, especially antiplatelet agents, antihypertensive drugs, and cholesterol-lowering agents. Nevertheless, the risk of vascular problems is considered higher in underlying atherosclerosis, which is why, in these cases, in addition to lifestyle modification and medication, regular follow-up examinations, especially using ultrasound, are necessary.

77. ***When does a leg have to be amputated in the case of a vascular occlusion?***

Amputation of the leg, medically referred to as leg amputation, is and remains an absolute exception. It should be reserved for cases in which the damage to the leg is so severe that preservation is not promising. This is always the case when the leg can no longer be expected to bear weight, for example, in the event of massive damage to muscle and nerve tissue. However, if the entire foot is filled with pus, amputation may also be unavoidable. A collection of pus is medically termed an abscess. This can particularly affect diabetics, who are at risk of developing extensive and deep abscesses. In the case of an abscess, there is not only the danger that the leg will be increasingly damaged, but also that infectious agents and waste products will be transported away by the blood, potentially causing blood poisoning.

If advanced vascular calcification (atherosclerosis) is present, amputation may also become necessary in the case of increasing pain or non-healing and progressively enlarging wounds. This particularly affects patients in whom an improvement in blood flow is not or no longer possible, and consequently, amputation is the last resort. Otherwise, in such cases, there would be a slow death of the leg, which could also lead to blood poisoning and, without amputation, can be fatal.

78. ***Are regular follow-up examinations important to prevent a renewed vascular occlusion?***

In principle, regular medical check-ups are recommended after every vascular occlusion. This is especially important in the case of vascular stenoses, to prevent a renewed occlusion due to increasing narrowing. During follow-up examinations, an ultrasound examination is usually performed, blood values are determined, and, if necessary, blood flow measurements are taken. In the event of increasing narrowing or other problems, an imaging examination is usually carried out, for example, a computed tomography or magnetic resonance angiography. Regular consultations with a specialist in heart diseases are also recommended after an arterial occlusion, especially if cardiac arrhythmias were the cause of the occlusion. However, in the case of vascular calcifications, cardiac examinations are also necessary, primarily to detect and treat coronary artery stenoses in a timely manner.

Stroke

79. ***My mother died of a stroke, how high is my risk of having one as well?***

This question cannot be answered in general terms. A stroke can result from cardiac arrhythmias, as well as from vascular calcification in the context of atherosclerosis, and ultimately also from a cerebral hemorrhage. Cardiac arrhythmias, especially atrial fibrillation, are heart conditions that become increasingly common with advancing age. There is also a familial predisposition, but age is usually the main risk factor. In atherosclerosis, the risk of having a stroke is increased. In addition to the typical risk factors for atherosclerosis (high blood pressure, elevated blood lipid levels, diabetes), there is also a familial clustering of vascular calcification. If the stroke is caused by a cerebral hemorrhage, it is often preceded by an accident, but sometimes also by high blood pressure or a so-called hypertensive crisis.

In summary, it can be said that there can indeed be a familial predisposition to stroke, but this is not always the case. Thus, a stroke in the family does not necessarily mean that you will also have one or that you are at high risk. Nevertheless, it is advisable to see a cardiologist for a heart examination and to have the carotid arteries examined by a vascular surgeon.

80. ***Why is a stroke colloquially called "Schlägle"?***

Especially in southern Germany, the term "Schlägle" is used for a "minor" stroke. Physicians refer to a "minor" stroke when it is a so-called TIA. The abbreviation stands for "transient ischemic attack" and refers to a temporary disturbance of blood flow to the brain. However, a TIA is a very serious condition and should always be treated with the utmost caution. A TIA can always develop into a full-blown stroke with permanent damage. Therefore, the seemingly harmless term "Schlägle" should be used with great caution. A "Schlägle" should always be seen as a warning sign and a precursor to the risk of suffering a real stroke.

S. Regus, *Answering Patients' Questions About Vascular Medicine*,
https://doi.org/10.1007/978-3-662-72771-3_8

81. ***Is stroke more common than heart attack?***

Strokes and heart attacks are the most common vascular diseases in Germany, often with very serious and severe consequences and complications. Each occurs at about the same frequency, with approximately 280,000 events per year.

In strokes, a distinction is made between those caused by a circulatory disorder (ischemic) and those caused by bleeding (hemorrhagic). With about 85%, circulatory disorders are the most common cause; this is referred to as an ischemic stroke. These circulatory disorders usually result from vascular calcification or an embolus originating from the heart due to arrhythmias. Brain hemorrhages, on the other hand, are usually caused by high blood pressure, a ruptured aneurysm in the brain, or a severe accident. This is then called a hemorrhagic stroke.

In summary, both stroke and heart attack can be serious complications of circulatory disorders and occur at roughly the same frequency. Cardiologists and cardiac surgeons are responsible for heart attacks, while neurologists and vascular surgeons are the specialists for treating strokes.

82. ***Is vascular calcification also the main cause of stroke?***

A stroke is a sudden disturbance of brain function. This can occur in the presence of a vascular disease either due to bleeding (too much blood) or a circulatory disorder (too little blood). In the case of bleeding, healthy brain tissue is displaced; this type of stroke is also called hemorrhagic. In the case of a circulatory disorder, also known as an ischemic stroke, there is a reduced supply of oxygen- and nutrient-rich blood. Most commonly (in about 80%), this is caused by an embolus, usually a blood clot from the heart, which becomes lodged in a cerebral artery and blocks it. Less commonly (in about 20%), ischemic stroke is caused by a narrowing of a carotid artery, which is usually due to vascular calcification (atherosclerosis). In this case, clots also form, but not in the heart; rather, they form at the site of the narrowed artery and are carried to the brain, where they trigger the stroke (see Fig. 1a–e).

Consequently, vascular calcification also plays a major role in stroke, but it is not the main cause of this condition.

83. ***Why should I have my carotid artery operated on even though I have no symptoms?***

Even if you have no symptoms, in selected cases, a preventive (prophylactic) operation for a narrowed carotid artery may be reasonable and recommended. This is particularly the case if the narrowing (stenosis) is increasing and exceeds 80%, or if the narrowing carries a high risk of clot formation that could be carried to the brain by the bloodstream. The greater the narrowing (degree of stenosis) and the higher the risk that parts of the vessel wall could detach from the narrowed area, the higher the risk of stroke. Consequently, surgery on the carotid artery is often a preventive procedure in a (still) asymptomatic patient to prevent a stroke. Of course, complications can also occur during surgery, potentially resulting in a

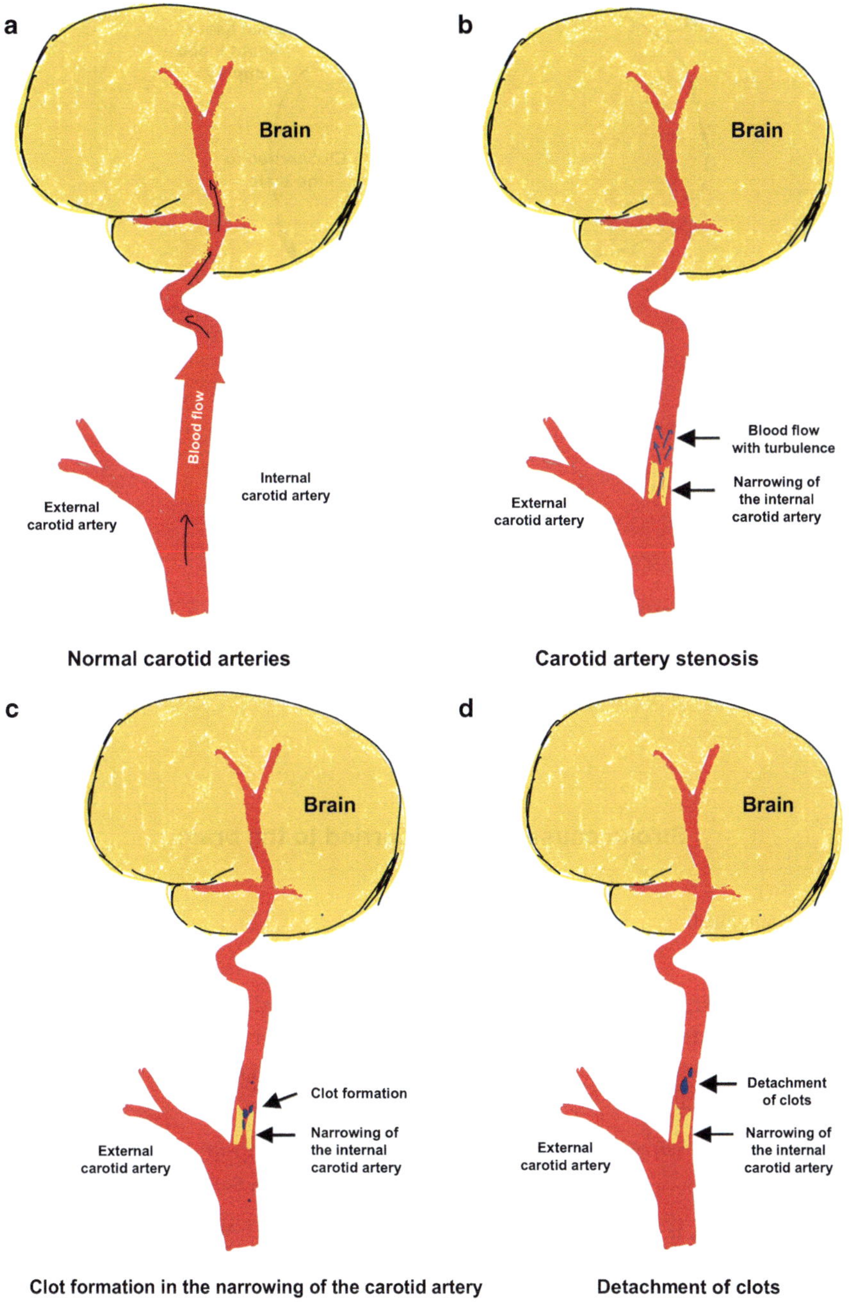

Fig. 1 (**a**) Normal flow conditions in a carotid artery, (**b**) Narrowing at the origin of the internal carotid artery with turbulence of blood flow, (**c**) Clot formation at the narrowing, (**d**) Detachment of the clot and embolization to the brain, (**e**) Stroke caused by an embolus in the brain

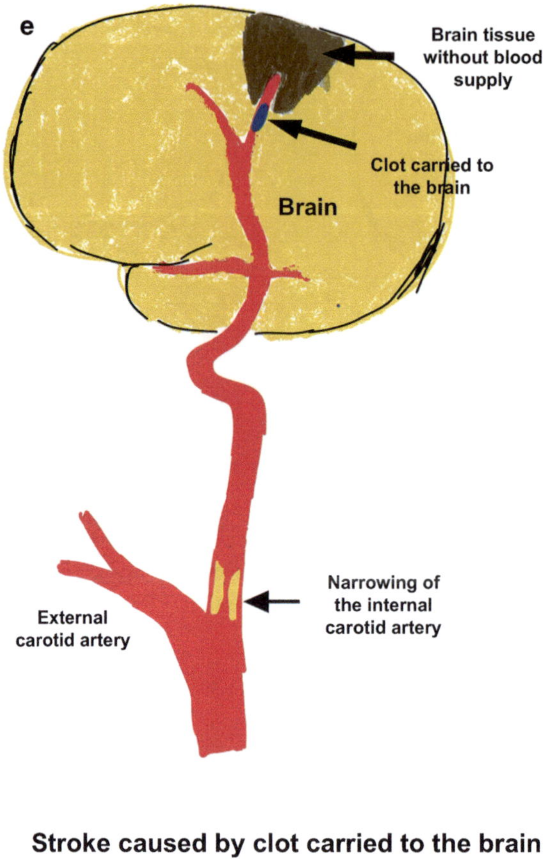

Fig. 1 (continued)

stroke. However, from a certain degree of stenosis onward, the risk of stroke if the narrowing is left untreated is higher than without surgery. Therefore, it may be that you are recommended to undergo carotid artery surgery even though you have no symptoms at all.

84. ***Why is my carotid artery not being operated on, even though it is 50% narrowed?***

If the narrowing is 50% or less, the risk of stroke is very low. In these cases, surgery is generally not recommended, as the risk of stroke from the operation is higher than if the narrowing is left untreated. However, if you have already had a minor stroke, the symptoms of which have completely resolved, surgery may sometimes be recommended even with a 50% narrowing. The minor stroke, also known as a transient ischemic attack (TIA), is considered a warning sign of a major stroke and should always be taken very seriously. Even—and especially—if the symptoms lasted only briefly and have completely disappeared, the problems can recur, and then a severe stroke may occur. For this reason, even with a moderate (50%) narrowing, surgery may be recommended as a preventive measure against a full-blown stroke.

85. *How is a narrowed carotid artery operated on?*

There are several ways to treat a narrowed carotid artery. One is the **conservative** approach, involving blood pressure management and administration of blood-thinning medications. In addition, there is surgery, in which the narrowed carotid artery is opened and the calcified plaque is removed. Finally, it is also possible to use a stent to widen the narrowed carotid artery.

During surgery, the carotid artery is exposed through an incision in the neck, opened, and the narrowing is removed. However, the carotid artery must be clamped for this, and sometimes a plastic tube, medically referred to as a shunt, is inserted (see Fig. 2). This may be necessary if blood flow to the brain is insufficient during the clamping phase. Therefore, during the operation, the function of the brain and especially cerebral blood flow are continuously monitored.

After the artery is cut at an angle, it can be turned inside out and the calcified narrowing removed. The technical term for this is "eversion endarterectomy." This is particularly useful if the vessel is too long and curves, as this surgical technique also allows the artery to be shortened and then sewn straight onto the original artery (see Fig. 3).

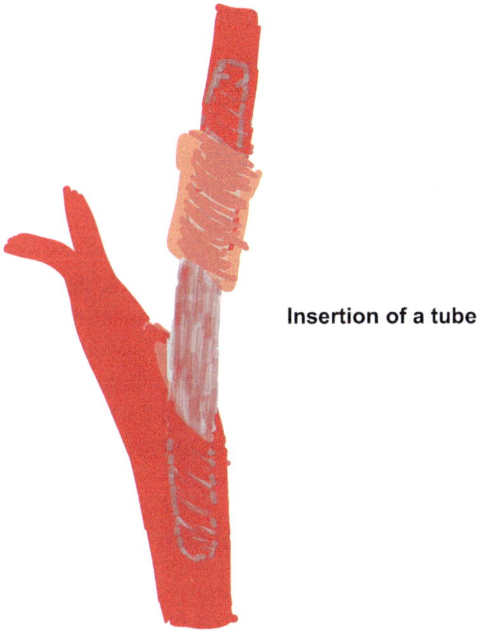

Fig. 2 Insertion of a tube (medically called a shunt) to ensure blood flow to the brain during surgery

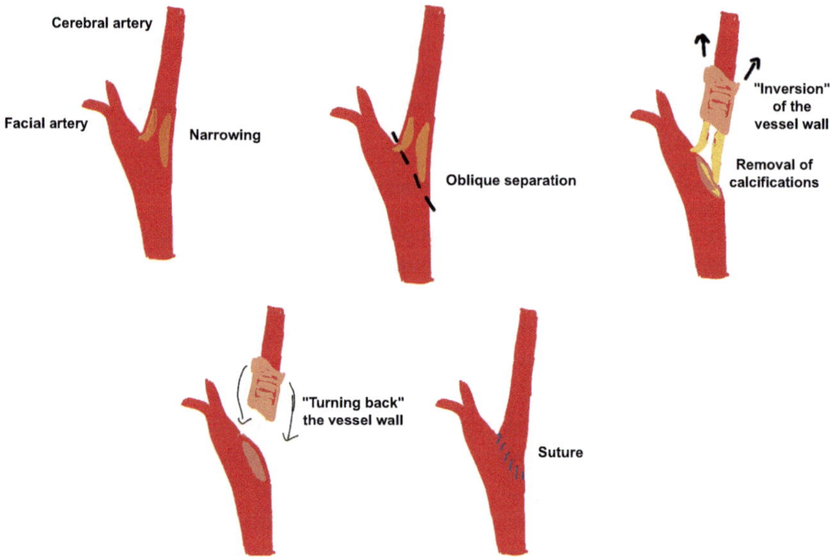

Fig. 3 Principle of surgery for a carotid artery stenosis using eversion endarterectomy

However, if the narrowed carotid artery is already very straight and elongated, it must be opened lengthwise, the calcified plaque removed, and a patch sewn in (medically called patch angioplasty).

86. ***How and when is a stent used?***

In stent treatment, a catheter is inserted through the femoral artery and advanced to the carotid artery. Once the narrowing is passed, it is dilated and a stent is placed.

Surgery therefore requires an incision to expose and remove the narrowing from the outside. With stenting, the narrowing is treated from the inside, requiring vascular access via the groin. The advantage of a stent is that no general anesthesia (except for local anesthesia at the groin) is needed and there is no surgical wound. The disadvantage of a stent is that advancing the catheter can dislodge clots from the narrowing, potentially causing a stroke. While this can also happen during surgery, the risk is usually lower. Nevertheless, there are cases in which a stent is recommended. These include, for example, patients who have already undergone surgery and have developed a new narrowing over time. In such cases, the risk of vascular and nerve injury during surgery is significantly increased due to scarring.

87. ***I am always dizzy—could this be due to my narrowed carotid artery?***

Dizziness is not a typical sign of a narrowed carotid artery, but rather suggests blood pressure problems, heart failure, or metabolic disorders (for example, blood sugar that is too high or too low). Narrowings of the cerebellar arteries can also cause dizziness, but these are much less common than carotid artery stenoses.

The majority of patients with carotid artery stenosis have no symptoms until a stroke occurs. The most common signs of a stroke are unilateral arm or leg weakness, speech disturbances, or temporary visual disturbances in one eye. A drooping corner of the mouth can also be a sign of a stroke. Dizziness is not a typical sign of a stroke.

88. ***Can I have a stroke during the operation?***

The purpose of surgery for a narrowed carotid artery is to prevent a stroke. In this procedure, the carotid artery is opened and the narrowed section, including the calcifications, is removed (see Fig. 4).

However, during the exposure of the carotid artery, there is a risk that clots from the narrowed section may be dislodged and travel to the brain, potentially causing a stroke. Fortunately, this is very rare. But even after the carotid artery has been opened and the narrowed section removed, a stroke can be triggered by the dislodgement of tiny fragments of the vessel wall once the artery is reopened to blood flow. Furthermore, a stroke can also occur during the phase when the carotid artery is clamped and the narrowing is being removed.

Overall, the risk of stroke during surgery is about 1–5%, which is significantly lower than if the narrowing is left untreated.

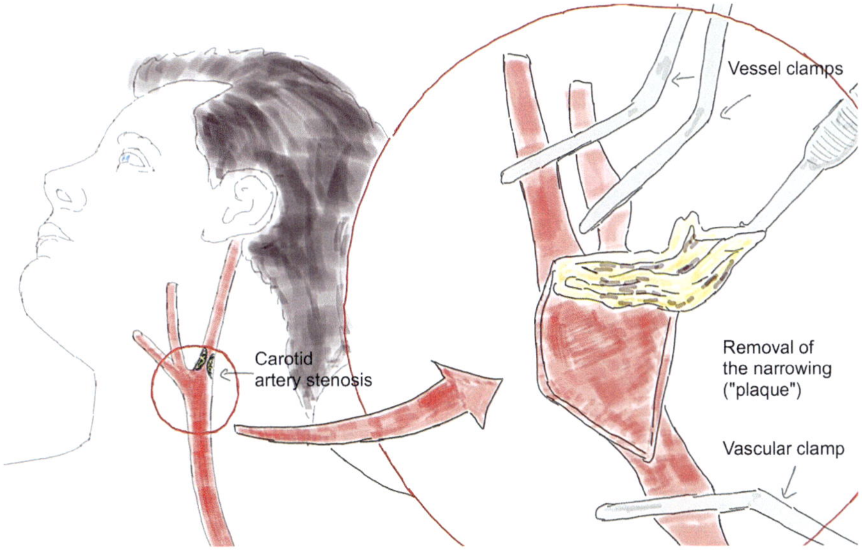

Fig. 4 Schematic representation of a carotid artery operation, in which the vessel is clamped and the plaque is removed

89. ***When is it advisable to undergo rehabilitation before the planned surgery following a stroke?***

A rehabilitation program is usually carried out after major or complex surgeries. This also includes surgery for a narrowed carotid artery, especially if a stroke has occurred beforehand or during or after the operation. Consequently, the treatment commonly referred to as "rehab" is also known as follow-up treatment.

However, if a major stroke has already occurred before the operation, it is often recommended to first undergo rehabilitation and then perform surgery on the narrowed carotid artery to eliminate the cause of the stroke. The reason for this is that surgery performed immediately after a severe stroke can lead to bleeding in the brain, which may cause another stroke and significantly worsen the patient's condition. Therefore, a recent and major stroke is a situation in which immediate carotid artery surgery should only be performed in exceptional cases and after thorough preliminary examination and assessment.

Aortic Aneurysm

90. ***What is an aortic aneurysm?***

An aortic aneurysm refers to a bulging (medically: aneurysm) of the main artery (medically: aorta). The normal diameter of the aorta is approximately 1.5–2 cm; an aneurysm is diagnosed when the diameter reaches 3 cm or more. The majority of aortic aneurysms affect the abdominal aorta below the diaphragm, most commonly below the origin of the renal arteries (see Fig. 1). Only 15–20% of aortic aneurysms are located above the diaphragm in the chest.

91. ***Why does an aortic aneurysm develop?***

An aortic aneurysm often develops as a result of vascular calcification (atherosclerosis), but it can also be caused by congenital (genetic) connective tissue disorders. Fundamentally, a reduction in vascular elasticity is considered the main cause for the formation of vascular bulges in the sense of aneurysm development. Smoking plays a decisive role as a risk factor for the development of atherosclerosis. The vast majority of patients with an aortic aneurysm caused by calcification are active smokers or have had a long history of nicotine abuse.

92. ***Why is it not necessary to operate on every aneurysm?***

Many patients with an aortic aneurysm have no symptoms at all. Therefore, the diagnosis of an aortic aneurysm is often made incidentally, for example, when an abdominal ultrasound is performed for other reasons. A typical scenario is also the investigation of back pain by MRI, during which parts of the abdominal aorta are imaged.

An aneurysm of the abdominal aorta should be operated on when the risk of rupture (risk of bursting) is increased. This risk rises with increasing diameter of the abdominal aorta and, at a diameter of 5.5 cm, is about 1–5% per year. Surgery is recommended from this diameter onward, as the risk of complications during surgery is lower than the risk of rupture.

S. Regus, *Answering Patients' Questions About Vascular Medicine*,
https://doi.org/10.1007/978-3-662-72771-3_9

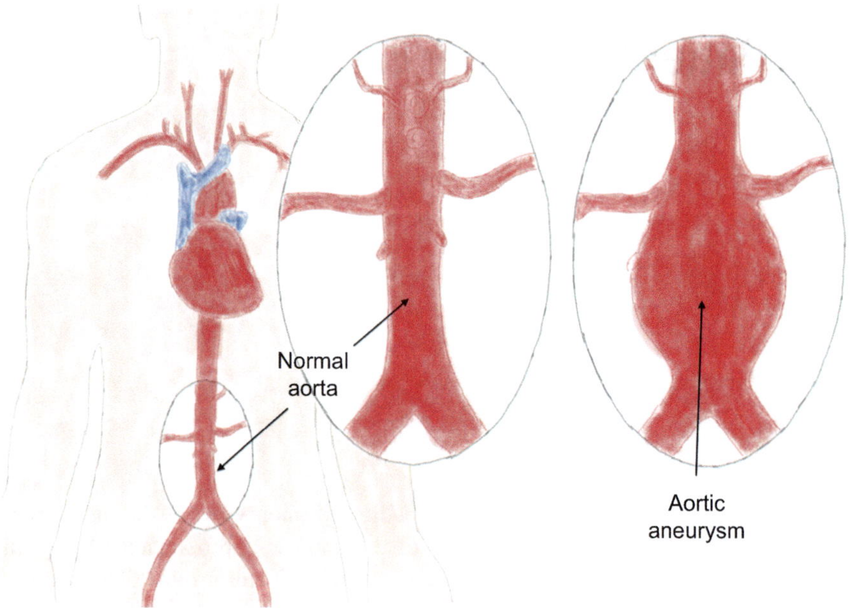

Fig. 1 Schematic representation of a normal abdominal aorta and a bulging, i.e., an aortic aneurysm

Regardless of diameter, any aneurysm that causes symptoms (most commonly pain) or increases rapidly in size should be treated.

An aneurysm that causes no symptoms and is smaller than 5 cm should be monitored regularly, usually by ultrasound examinations. The risk of rupture is very low in this case and is less than the risk of complications during surgery.

93. ***Why does my aneurysm need to be operated on?***

The recommendation to have an aneurysm surgically treated will be made by your attending physician. Normally, the indication for surgery is given when the aneurysm is sufficiently large or is causing symptoms. Of course, a ruptured aneurysm also constitutes an indication for surgery, but the chances of survival in this situation are very low. On average, only one in ten patients with a ruptured aneurysm reaches the hospital alive and can undergo surgery. However, only half of these patients survive the operation. Therefore, an aneurysm should be operated on whenever possible before it ruptures.

As already explained in detail, both a diameter of 5.5 cm and an increase in size of 1 cm per year are indications for surgery.

94. ***What happens if I do not have surgery?***

If the aneurysm is still below the diameter at which surgery is recommended, regular follow-up examinations are performed, usually by ultrasound. If the diameter increases to over 5.5 cm, surgery is generally recommended. However, if surgery is not performed—either because the patient does not wish it or because, for example, the anesthesia risk is too high—there is a risk that the aneurysm will rupture. This risk increases with increasing diameter. If the aneurysm ruptures, the patient may bleed to death internally immediately. This occurs if the aneurysm ruptures freely into the abdominal cavity and all the blood flows into the abdomen within seconds. However, if the aneurysm ruptures to the side or backward toward the spine (this space is called the retroperitoneum, i.e., located behind the abdominal cavity), most patients experience abdominal and back pain and may feel dizzy or lose consciousness. Since the retroperitoneum is much smaller than the abdominal cavity, patients usually do not bleed to death immediately and can reach the hospital alive. Further treatment, including surgery, can then be provided. If a patient refuses aneurysm surgery, this applies both in the case of a non-ruptured and a ruptured aneurysm. In both situations, the patient's wishes should be respected, especially in the case of rupture, when the patient is usually no longer responsive or able to communicate and thus cannot express their wishes. It is important that this information is communicated to the emergency physicians. In this case, transport to the hospital can be omitted, as this is in accordance with the patient's wishes.

95. ***Which is better: surgery via the groin or through the abdomen?***

This cannot be answered in general terms. The operation via the groin is, in principle, smaller and less stressful for the body, as only a small incision is made in the groin or the vessel is punctured through the skin with large needles (see Fig. 2). This surgical procedure is also referred to as minimally invasive (because only skin incisions in the groin are necessary) or endovascular (because the exclusion of the aneurysm is performed from the inside). The principle of the operation via the groin is to advance a stent graft from this point under X-ray guidance into the aneurysm. The stent graft (also called endoprosthesis, because it is inserted and

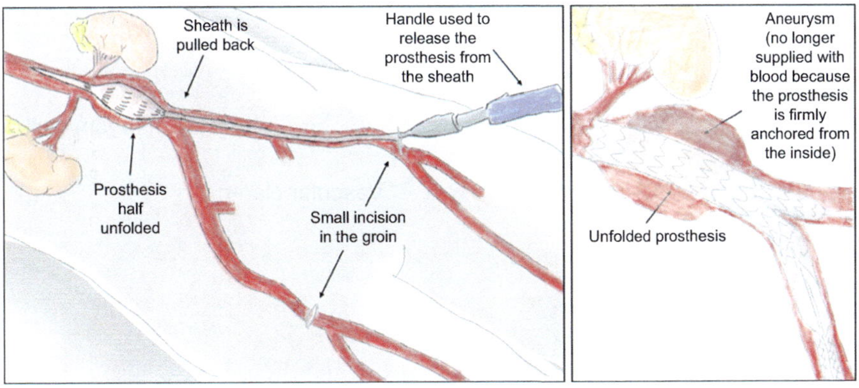

Fig. 2 Principle of endovascular exclusion of an aortic aneurysm via the femoral arteries

deployed from the inside) is contained in a sheath about the thickness of a pencil and unfolds as soon as the sheath is withdrawn. The stent graft consists of metal (stent) and a synthetic covering (graft). However, this stent graft (or endoprosthesis) must unfold in such a way that it can anchor itself securely above and below the aneurysm. In this way, the aneurysm is, so to speak, splinted from the inside and rupture is prevented.

In the operation via the abdomen, the entire abdomen is opened and the aneurysm is exposed (see Fig. 3).

In this procedure, blood loss can be significantly higher than with the operation via the groin, and postoperative pain is often much greater than with the groin approach.

However, problems can also arise during the operation via the groin that necessitate opening the abdomen. In addition, after the operation, regular follow-up examinations via the groin are necessary, which are not necessarily required after open surgery. These follow-up examinations are necessary because leaks in the prosthesis occur more frequently after the operation via the groin, which then also need to be treated over time. Therefore, the decision as to whether the open or endovascular approach via the groin is chosen must always be made individually and after thorough patient counseling. The shape of the aneurysm also plays a role, as not every aneurysm can be treated endovascularly.

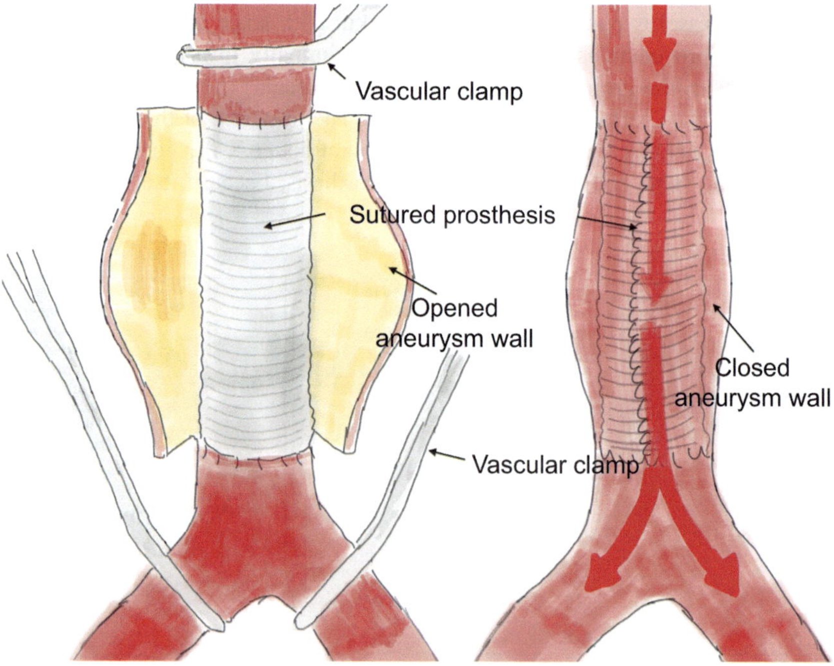

Fig. 3 Principle of open exclusion of an aortic aneurysm after opening the abdominal cavity

96. ***Is the endovascular operation via the groin performed under general anesthesia?***

Compared to the operation via the abdomen, the operation via the groin can also be performed under local anesthesia. However, this requires the patient to remain still, which can sometimes be difficult. Therefore, many patients require sedatives, especially if, for example, back pain makes it difficult to lie still for a longer period. Depending on the complexity of the operation, it can last from 30 minutes to several hours. Normally, the patient can decide for themselves which type of anesthesia they prefer in this case. However, spinal anesthesia is generally not used, as the risk of bleeding into the spinal canal is too high and damage to the spinal cord up to paraplegia can occur.

For anxious patients, general anesthesia is certainly the best option and nowadays can be performed gently in the vast majority of cases.

97. ***Is there anything I can do to make the aneurysm shrink again?***

The only way to make an aneurysm shrink is surgical treatment with a stent graft. When the aneurysm is splinted from the inside by the graft, the pressure in the aneurysm sac decreases and it becomes smaller over time (see Fig. 4a–c).

One can imagine it like a soccer ball that gradually loses air over time, causing the pressure to decrease. Although the soccer ball does not change its size, it becomes flat due to the drop in pressure (see Fig. 5a, b).

Without surgery, the aneurysm will, at best, remain the same size, but it will not get smaller. To minimize the risk of the aneurysm increasing in size, risk factors such as high blood pressure and asthma should be well controlled, and smoking should be stopped. While this is no guarantee that the aneurysm will shrink or remain small, it is at least the only way for patients to exert some influence.

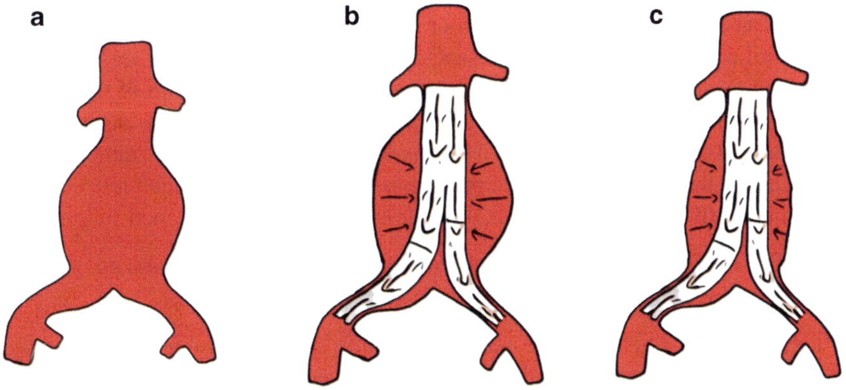

Fig. 4 (**a**) Untreated and fully pressurized aneurysm, (**b**) Aneurysm shortly after exclusion by endoprosthesis, still filled but no longer under pressure, (**c**) Aneurysm sac shrinks some time after treatment

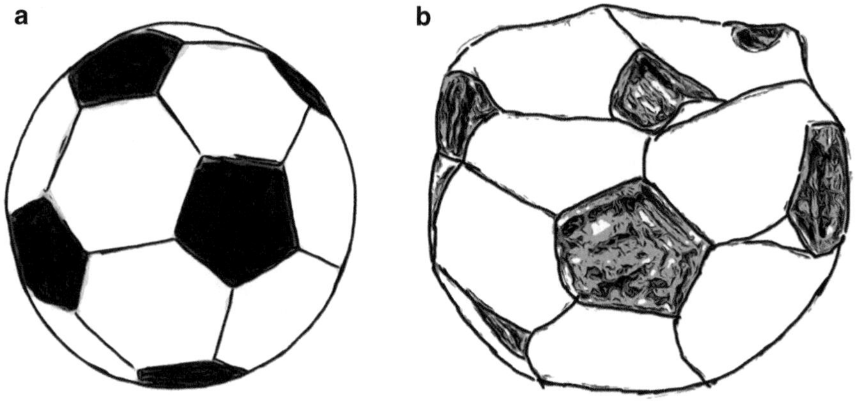

Fig. 5 (**a**) Fully inflated soccer ball, (**b**) Flat soccer ball lacking air and therefore pressure

To monitor the success of the above-mentioned risk factor management, regular ultrasound examinations are performed. The primary purpose is to monitor whether the aneurysm remains stable or increases in size.

98. ***How great is my risk that the aneurysm will rupture?***

The risk of rupture (i.e., bursting) depends on the size and growth rate of the aneurysm. With a diameter of less than 5 cm, the risk is about 1% per year. As the diameter increases, the risk rises rapidly and reaches 30–50% per year at 8 cm. Abdominal or back pain for which there is no other cause than the aneurysm is also associated with a higher risk of rupture. In these cases, it is referred to as a symptomatic aneurysm, meaning one that is already causing pain and thus represents an urgent indication for surgery.

99. ***Can the aneurysm still rupture after a stent has been placed?***

If the stent is not properly positioned or becomes loose over time, a rupture of the aneurysm can occur despite the presence of the stent graft. For this reason, regular follow-up examinations should be performed to check the position of the prosthesis and to rule out any leaks. After open surgery, a rupture can also occur, but not at the site of the aneurysm, since it has been removed beforehand; rather, the tear can occur at the suture sites of the prosthesis. However, this is much less common, so significantly fewer follow-up examinations are required after open surgery.

100. ***Do I need to have regular follow-up examinations if I do not undergo surgery?***

If the aneurysm is not yet large enough to require surgery, regular follow-up examinations, usually by ultrasound, should be performed. Depending on the size and appearance of the aneurysm, these are carried out every 3–6 months.

However, if the aneurysm is already so large that surgery is recommended but the patient refuses, further follow-up examinations are generally no longer indicated. If the patient refuses surgery, it is usually a fundamental refusal—both in the asymptomatic stage and, even more so, in the event of rupture. This should be discussed in detail with the patient and their relatives and documented accordingly. The relatives and the patient should also be informed that, in the event of a rupture, hospital transport should not be arranged. Rather, if emergency services are contacted at all, the emergency personnel should be informed of the situation and the patient's refusal of surgery.

101. ***And what if I do have surgery?***

If the operation is performed via the groin with an endoprosthesis ("stent"), then regular follow-up examinations are essential. After open surgery, follow-up examinations are also often performed, but these are generally less frequent and not strictly necessary if the findings in the initial period after surgery are unremarkable.

102. ***What follow-up examinations are necessary?***

After surgery with an endoprosthesis ("stent"), follow-up examinations usually require CT scans; if the course is unremarkable, ultrasound may also be used.

For open surgery via abdominal incision, clinical examinations are generally sufficient, in which the condition of the scars is checked and the abdominal wall is palpated for softness. In addition, the suture sites of the prosthesis can be checked by ultrasound, which can be omitted over time if the findings remain unremarkable.

Since a large proportion of patients with an aortic aneurysm have so-called cardiovascular risk factors—such as high blood pressure, diabetes, elevated blood values, and smoking—follow-up examinations should also include risk factor reduction, especially smoking cessation. Due to these risk factors, many patients also have changes in the coronary arteries, which can lead to heart attack. Therefore, follow-up examinations of the heart and coronary arteries are also necessary, usually by cardiac ultrasound and ECG.

103. ***Do I have to take blood thinners?***

As a rule, blood thinning is not necessary solely because of the aneurysm. However, since the majority of aneurysms are due to atherosclerosis, a so-called platelet inhibitor is usually prescribed. This is a medication that prevents blood platelets (thrombocytes) from clumping together, thereby reducing the risk of clot formation.

Stronger blood thinning, e.g., with Marcumar®, is rarely necessary because of the aneurysm itself, but rather for cardiological reasons (for example, due to heart conditions).

104. ***When can I return to work after the operation?***

This depends on which operation was performed. As a rule, after endovascular surgery via the groin, it is possible to return to work sooner. The hospital stay is also usually much shorter than with open surgery. However, there are no rules that apply to all patients, and the patient's own perception, ability to recover, and fitness before the procedure are also decisive for resilience. Most patients are able to return to work within 2 weeks after groin-based surgery, and after open surgery via abdominal incision, after about 4–6 weeks. However, these time frames only apply if the operation and postoperative course were uneventful.

105. ***Can I exert myself and play sports, even if I do not have surgery?***

An abdominal aortic aneurysm is not a contraindication for sports or physical activity. In particular, a small aneurysm that does not yet require surgery does not have, or at most only a negligibly higher, risk of rupture due to sports or exertion.

Even larger aneurysms that would require surgery due to their diameter are not a reason to stop exercising. On the contrary, sports and a healthy lifestyle can help halt the underlying atherosclerosis that causes aneurysms. In other words: sports and quitting smoking can slow the growth of aneurysms, but cannot reverse the aneurysm itself.

106. ***Why isn't every aneurysm treated with a stent?***

Surgery with a stent is not possible in some cases, especially if it cannot be properly anchored. Above and below the aneurysm, the stent graft must be able to anchor securely without blocking important arterial branches. These important branches from the main abdominal artery (aorta) include, for example, arteries supplying the kidneys (renal arteries) or the intestines and liver (mesenteric arteries). A severe kink in the vessels above or below the bulge can also make stent graft placement difficult. In addition, very narrow pelvic vessels are sometimes a reason why open surgery is recommended. This is because the prostheses must be advanced through the pelvic arteries up into the abdominal or thoracic aorta, which can be difficult with very thin arteries.

However, due to advances in stent graft technology, open surgery is becoming increasingly rare. For example, there are prostheses that are custom-made for each patient and have special openings for arterial branches or small side branches through which the vessels can then be supplied.

107. ***Can the stent operation also be performed on an outpatient basis?***

The so-called minimally invasive endovascular treatment of an aortic aneurysm is less invasive, and therefore usually significantly less stressful than open surgery. Nevertheless, outpatient treatment is not possible or not recommended. This is because, even with this operation, anesthesia is often necessary, postoperative pain may occur, or complications may arise. For example, fever may develop after the operation if an infection occurs or if the body reacts to the foreign material of the prosthesis. These episodes of fever, accompanied by a pronounced feeling of illness, can occur for several days after the operation and usually resolve on their own. Nevertheless, inpatient monitoring is sensible and recommended in these cases. The situation is different for stent implantations in the pelvic region. These procedures can be performed on an outpatient basis. However, even in these cases, complications such as bleeding at the groin puncture sites can occur, which is why home care must be ensured. This means that someone must pick up the patient from the clinic and ensure that they are present at home. This is particularly important in case complications arise and an emergency readmission to the hospital becomes necessary.

108. ***What would you recommend to me: open or endovascular surgery?***

To answer this question, some important information must first be obtained:

1. What does the aneurysm look like, and in particular, what is the condition of the healthy sections of the aorta above and below it?

This is important in order to decide whether internal stenting is possible and promising. The decisive factor here is whether the so-called landing zones are sufficiently long so that a prosthesis can be anchored there and seal off the aneurysm. If the landing zones are too short, open surgery should be considered.

2. Are there calcifications or narrowings of the iliac arteries?

If the pelvic arteries are calcified and too narrow, it can be difficult to advance a prosthesis and place it in the aneurysm. In some cases, this can be achieved by balloon dilation and stenting. Long-segment stenoses or occlusions of the iliac arteries are problematic.

3. Has the patient previously undergone abdominal surgery?

This may favor an endovascular approach, as repeat interventions (i.e., procedures after previous surgeries) in the abdomen are significantly more difficult and associated with an increased risk of complications.

4. What is the surgical and anesthesia risk?

Patients with severe pre-existing conditions, especially heart and lung diseases, often benefit from an endovascular approach. This is because this surgical technique is often faster, less invasive, and associated with less blood loss.

5. How old is the patient?

Younger and healthier patients can also be recommended open surgery, as there is no radiation exposure during the operation. Open surgery is performed without X-ray imaging, as the surgeon is directly on site and exposes and visualizes the aneurysm. In addition, with open surgery, regular follow-up with computed tomography is not necessary, which would otherwise lead to radiation exposure.

6. Is the patient male?

In men, it must always be mentioned during the informed consent discussion for open surgery that problems with potency may occur. This is because important nerves in front of the aorta, which are essential for erection and ejaculation, can be injured during open surgery. Therefore, it may be the explicit wish of sexually active men to undergo endovascular surgery via the femoral arteries.

109. ***Is an aortic aneurysm a common disease?***

Overall, the aortic aneurysm is a rare disease, with a prevalence of about 1% worldwide. This means that an estimated one in a hundred people is affected. However, younger people are rarely affected, whereas the likelihood increases with age. In the age group between 65 and 85 years, the prevalence is already 4–5%, with men being affected six times more often than women. Therefore, all men and all at-risk women with relevant risk factors (nicotine abuse, high blood pressure, diabetes mellitus, known vascular diseases in the family) are recommended to have an ultrasound examination from the age of 50 in order to detect or rule out an aortic aneurysm at an early stage. Even though it is a rare disease, complications can be fatal and could be prevented by early treatment.

110. ***Is an aortic aneurysm hereditary?***

There are different causes of an aortic aneurysm, including a congenital predisposition. This is also referred to as familial clustering of aneurysms, as these are passed down from generation to generation through a defective gene (or several). However, this form of aneurysm is much less common than those caused by atherosclerosis (vascular wall calcification). The latter is caused by risk factors such as smoking, high blood pressure, or diabetes mellitus.

In familial aortic aneurysms, it is typical for the aneurysms to occur at a younger age, whereas the more common form associated with atherosclerosis is usually discovered at an older age. Thus, it is not uncommon for the aneurysm to occur (sometimes well) before the age of 30 in cases of familial predisposition, while the atherosclerotic aneurysm is usually detected between the ages of 50 and 60.

111. ***Can you feel it if you have an aortic aneurysm?***

In most cases, patients do not feel that they have an aortic aneurysm. Occasionally, a pulsating mass, that is, a swelling pulsating with the heartbeat, can be palpated at the level of the navel. However, since most people are not aware that such a swelling and pulsation can be caused by an aortic aneurysm, the aneurysm often remains undetected even in these cases. This can become dangerous if the aneurysm increases in size and, in the worst case, ruptures. Therefore, check-up examinations at the family doctor should also include ultrasound examinations of the abdomen and abdominal aorta to detect and monitor aneurysms at an early stage.

112. ***What examinations can be used to detect an aortic aneurysm?***

An aortic aneurysm in the abdominal region can be detected by palpation alone if it is large enough, whereas an aortic aneurysm in the chest area usually cannot be palpated.

The next important examination for investigating and detecting an aortic aneurysm is ultrasound. With this, the size and condition can often already be determined, although this examination technique is sometimes somewhat limited. This is because ultrasound cannot penetrate air-filled tissues, which is particularly problematic in the abdomen due to the intestines and in the chest due to the lungs.

The purpose of the ultrasound examination is to detect the aneurysm. More precise information about the size, structure, extent, and location of the aneurysm can subsequently be obtained with a computed tomography (CT) scan. Before surgery for an aortic aneurysm, a CT scan is routinely performed, especially prior to endovascular procedures involving a "stent." In these surgical techniques, it is essential to thoroughly assess the appearance of the aneurysm, and based on the CT scan, precisely fitting prostheses must then be ordered. However, even before "open surgical" procedures involving a large abdominal incision, a CT scan is generally performed, as this is the only way to determine which prosthesis—either one to be sewn in directly or one to be inserted via the groin—is most suitable for the patient.

113. ***How is an aortic aneurysm treated?***

There are three ways to treat an aortic aneurysm:

1. The first option is to regularly monitor and examine the aneurysm, prescribe medication, and recommend a healthy lifestyle. In particular, smoking should be avoided. This approach is also referred to as "**conservative**" management, as it does not involve surgery. It is especially recommended when the bulge is small and the rate of growth is low.
2. However, if the aneurysm reaches a size of more than 5 cm or increasingly causes problems (such as abdominal or back pain), an invasive procedure is recommended. "Invasive" means that the integrity of the body is breached from the outside in order to treat a disease. By using prostheses introduced via the groin, which are contained in a sheath and only expand once in place inside the body, the aneurysm can be sealed off. This is called an **endovascular** procedure, because the vessel (vascular) is sealed from the inside (endo). However, the prosthesis must anchor itself in the healthy artery above and below the aneurysm in order to seal it off. Since the prosthesis is introduced via the femoral artery, small incisions or even just punctures are usually sufficient.
3. In some cases, however, a prosthesis introduced via the groin may not anchor properly in the bulge (the aneurysm), in which case an **open operation** is recommended. In this procedure, the abdominal cavity is opened along its entire length and the aneurysm is removed. To restore blood flow, a prosthesis must be sewn in. This method is called open surgery, which is in principle possible for any aneurysm.

Kidney Failure and Dialysis

114. ***Why do I need a shunt?***

A shunt is always necessary when kidney function is so impaired that an artificial kidney is required. The latter refers to a device that cleans the blood, thereby removing metabolic waste products and excess electrolytes. This procedure is technically called hemodialysis, commonly referred to as blood washing. Hemodialysis takes about 3–4 hours and usually needs to be repeated three times a week. In order to withdraw blood from the body, either a catheter is needed, which is inserted through a vein in the neck or shoulder area. However, it is better to have a vessel located under the skin that can be punctured for dialysis. For this purpose, a shunt is created, ideally consisting of the patient's own vessels. The shunt should ensure a blood flow of at least 500 ml/min; otherwise, dialysis would take too long and occupy the entire day. This would be extremely uncomfortable for the patient and would further reduce the already diminished quality of life. The shunt is an artificial connection between an artery and a vein to achieve sufficient and appropriately high blood flow in the vein. In addition, the increased pressure coming from the artery causes the vein wall to thicken over the first few weeks, allowing the shunt to be punctured several times a week without any problems (see Fig. 1a, b).

115. ***Is the shunt visible from the outside?***

A shunt is not initially visible. It is usually located beneath the skin surface and is not exposed. However, what can be seen are enlargements of the shunt vein, which may develop over time. These enlargements are called aneurysms, caused by the increased pressure in the vein as well as the regular puncturing, medically referred to as puncture . The sites where the shunt is punctured may also become visible over time as scarred, altered streaks. Sometimes the skin over the shunt vein and the puncture sites may also become discolored. If a synthetic shunt has been placed, it can become infected and visible through the skin. In such cases, the shunt is also visible externally.

S. Regus, *Answering Patients' Questions About Vascular Medicine*,
https://doi.org/10.1007/978-3-662-72771-3_10

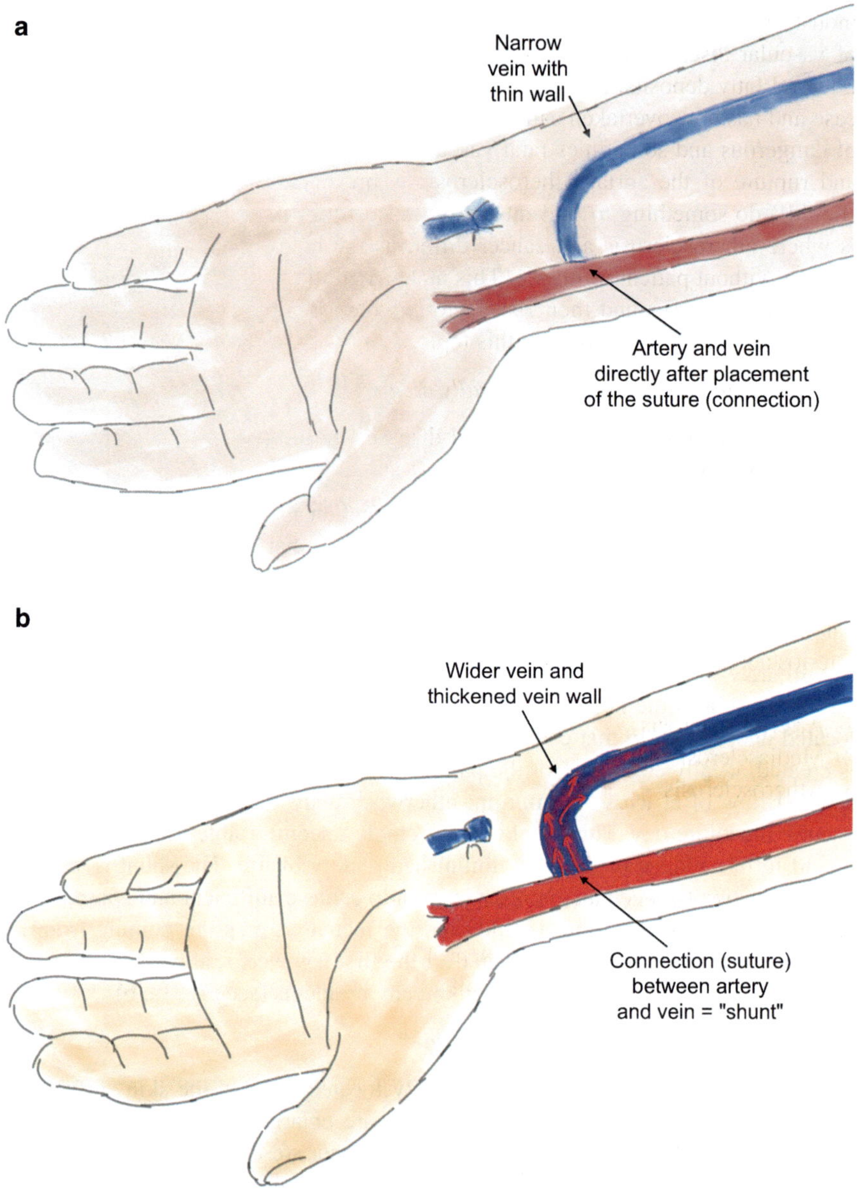

Fig. 1 (**a**) Typical finding after creating a connection between an artery and a vein (= shunt). The vein (blue) is still too thin to be punctured regularly. (**b**) Finding a few weeks after shunt creation. The vein wall has now thickened and the shunt vein can be punctured

116. ***Do I have to keep the shunt for life?***

How long a shunt is needed depends, among other things, on how severe the kidney damage is and how long it has existed. The cause of the kidney dysfunction also plays an important role. Stress, infections, or physical overexertion can cause temporary kidney dysfunction. Diabetes, genetic diseases such as polycystic kidney disease, or kidney damage from long-term use of painkillers often lead to severe impairment of kidney function that is irreversible. In such cases, the creation of a shunt is strongly recommended, as it has significantly fewer complications compared to a dialysis catheter and usually remains open and usable for a longer period. In cases of chronic renal insufficiency, which refers to kidney damage that does not recover, only a kidney transplant can provide relief and make the shunt unnecessary.

117. ***Why does my shunt close so often?***

If a shunt becomes occluded, there can be several causes. On the one hand, the inflow from the arteries may be too poor and too weak to maintain flow in the shunt. This can occur, for example, in the context of arterial occlusive disease, atherosclerosis. In such cases, dilation of the arteries or the creation of a new shunt is recommended. Furthermore, the outflow in the shunt may also be impaired, for example if the veins in the arm or chest are narrowed. Here, too, attempts can be made to dilate the narrowed vessels with balloon catheters. If in doubt, or if dilation is unsuccessful, the creation of a new shunt should be considered. Not infrequently, changes within the shunt itself, most commonly due to regular puncturing, are responsible for deterioration of shunt function or shunt occlusion.

118. ***How does a shunt actually work?***

The principle of a hemodialysis shunt is that a nearby artery is connected to a vein. The advantage of the artery is that blood is pumped out of the heart with strong pressure and therefore flows much more than in a vein. The special feature of veins, on the other hand, is that blood is transported back to the heart and flows much more slowly. However, veins are usually more superficial than arteries and can therefore be regularly punctured through the skin, which is essential for dialysis. Since normal veins have too little blood flow and the vein wall is too thin, successful blood washing cannot be performed through them. Hence the connection to the strong artery that transports much more blood. If the vein is too thin, it may be necessary to interpose a tubular synthetic graft.

119. ***Why can't the shunt be punctured immediately?***

A hemodialysis shunt requires a so-called maturation phase. This refers to the first few weeks after the connection between artery and vein is created, during which the vein changes due to the increased pressure (coming from the artery). It becomes thicker, larger, and especially the vein wall increases in thickness. After a few weeks, both the flow in the vein and the wall thickness are suitable for puncturing the shunt and performing hemodialysis through it. If the shunt is punctured too early, the vein wall may be damaged and a bruise (hematoma) may develop after the needle is removed. If a synthetic shunt is punctured too early, a hematoma may form around the shunt. In this case, the main issue is not the change in the shunt itself, but rather that the synthetic material must first grow into the tissue before it can be punctured.

120. ***Why do I need a catheter in my neck even though a shunt is also being created?***

A hemodialysis shunt can generally not be used immediately after placement. In most cases, several weeks must pass until the so-called "maturation phase" is complete and needling (referred to as puncture) is possible. The maturation phase refers to the period during which the shunt, after the connection between artery and vein has been established, undergoes changes such that the vein wall becomes thicker, the diameter increases, and puncture eventually becomes feasible. Ideally, the shunt is therefore created several weeks in advance, while hemodialysis is not yet necessary. However, kidney function can sometimes deteriorate so rapidly that the shunt cannot be placed early enough, and a catheter must be inserted in the neck as a temporary measure. This catheter can and should, however, be removed as soon as possible to prevent infection of the plastic tube and thrombosis of the vein.

121. ***Can I go home immediately after the shunt surgery?***

In most cases, the creation of a hemodialysis shunt can be performed on an outpatient basis. Preparation for the surgery takes place beforehand, and on the day of the operation, the patient usually must arrive fasting and may return home after a monitoring period of 1–2 hours. This is provided that the surgery went smoothly and the postoperative course was uneventful. It is also important that sufficient pain medication is available at home or has been obtained in advance. A follow-up check of the shunt is generally required a few days after the operation, which, depending on the attending physicians, can be performed by the surgeon, the general practitioner, or the dialysis doctors.

However, if it is a complex, i.e., more difficult shunt, inpatient monitoring may be necessary. More difficult shunts are to be expected, for example, when the vascular situation is very limited, the vessels are very thin, or multiple previous operations have already taken place. Existing dialysis dependency can also, in some cases, be a reason to perform the surgical procedure under inpatient conditions.

122. ***When should you see a vascular surgeon due to kidney insufficiency?***

Referral to vascular surgery usually occurs when the specialists in kidney diseases (nephrologists) can already foresee that dialysis will very likely be necessary. The role of the vascular surgeon in this situation is to perform special examinations such as ultrasound and blood flow measurements and to recommend which shunt should be placed and at which site. In some cases, dialysis via a catheter in the neck may also be necessary, but this should be avoided whenever possible. Ideally, referral to vascular surgery occurs early enough to create a shunt before dialysis becomes necessary. Conversely, a shunt should not be placed if dialysis will not be required afterwards. For this reason, close collaboration between vascular surgeons and nephrologists is extremely important for the continued successful treatment of patients with kidney disease and those requiring dialysis.

123. ***How many dialysis patients are there in Germany?***

The number of people with kidney disease is steadily increasing and currently stands at about 9 million in Germany. About half of these have chronic, i.e., permanent, kidney disease, and approximately 100,000 people depend on blood purification (dialysis). In principle, only a kidney transplant can provide a remedy here. However, the number of kidney transplants per year is lower than the number of new cases of patients requiring dialysis. This is because there are too few donor organs and, at the same time, the number of patients requiring dialysis increases from year to year.

124. ***Are there centers for dialysis shunts in children?***

The creation of dialysis shunts in children is demanding and requires a high level of surgical expertise. This is because children have thinner vessels, which typically contract (become spastic) when touched, making them even smaller. Therefore, creating the anastomoses (connections between artery and shunt vein) in children can be very challenging and, despite excellent suturing technique, can lead to immediate closure.

These problems can be reduced and the risk of shunt occlusion decreased not only through extensive surgical experience but also by using special instruments (microinstruments) and vasodilating medications.

It should be noted, however, that children suffer from the regularly necessary punctures of the dialysis shunt, as these can be very painful. Therefore, for very young and anxious children, it should be considered whether another, less painful dialysis method should be preferred. These include peritoneal dialysis or blood purification via a catheter. Parents can obtain details and individual advice on the most suitable approach at a pediatric dialysis center. Here, pediatricians, pediatric nephrologists, and vascular specialists work closely together to offer the affected child the best possible treatment.

125. ***What are the most common causes of dialysis dependency?***

The most common causes of kidney disease requiring blood purification, i.e., hemodialysis, are diabetes mellitus, untreated or poorly controlled high blood pressure (arterial hypertension), and congenital cystic diseases (polycystic kidney disease). Chronic use of painkillers can also damage the kidneys and lead to kidney failure. Ultimately, inflammation and malformations of the kidney or ureter, as well as the prostate gland, are also possible causes of chronic kidney insufficiency, which worsens over months and years.

Causes of sudden (acute) kidney dysfunction, also referred to as kidney failure, include circulatory shock, blood poisoning, or extreme fluid loss. In cases of acute kidney failure, blood purification is usually only required for a short period until the kidneys recover.

126. ***How can you tell if your kidneys are diseased?***

When kidney function is impaired, various problems—referred to as symptoms by medical professionals—can occur. These include fatigue, exhaustion, frequent or very infrequent urination, weight loss or gain, nausea, vomiting, and diarrhea. Skin changes are also common, including itching and very dry skin. The urine may be discolored, appear foamy, or contain blood. Cardiac arrhythmias may occur, and high blood pressure may be noticeable. Increased susceptibility to infections and anemia are also typical signs of impaired kidney function. An acute, i.e., sudden, reduction in kidney function up to complete failure is a very serious condition and always requires urgent hospital treatment.

127. ***Do you also receive all pre- and post-examinations of kidney function in vascular surgery?***

When a hemodialysis shunt is created, important examinations should be performed in vascular surgery beforehand. These are primarily examinations that relate to the surgical specifics of creating the hemodialysis shunt. In particular, the properties and course of the blood vessels are essential before placement. Afterwards, i.e., after the operation, special attention is paid to changes in the blood vessels following the creation of the connection between artery and vein. The flow in the shunt vein is of interest, as are the diameter and wall thickness. In vascular surgery, pre- and post-examinations therefore focus almost exclusively on the hemodialysis shunt. All functions relating to kidney function are generally assessed during dialysis and at follow-up appointments with the kidney specialist (nephrologist).

128. ***What examinations are necessary before shunt placement?***

Before creating a dialysis shunt, examinations to assess kidney function and the progression of dysfunction are first necessary. These provide information on whether the creation of a dialysis shunt is required and, in particular, when it should be performed. These examinations—usually laboratory tests and ultrasound examinations of the kidney—are almost exclusively carried out by specialists in kidney diseases (nephrologists). Specific examinations prior to the creation of a hemodialysis shunt from a vascular surgical perspective include ultrasound examinations of the vessels in the arm where the shunt is to be placed. Usually, the left arm is used in right-handed individuals (and conversely, the right arm in left-handed individuals). The key aspect of the ultrasound examinations is to determine whether the size of the vessels is sufficient and the blood flow is strong. This is important in order to determine whether, and especially at which site and level (forearm or upper arm), the shunt should be created. It can also be determined with a high degree of certainty whether the use of synthetic material will be necessary.

129. ***Why can't blood purification be performed permanently via a catheter in the neck?***

In principle, blood purification can also be performed for a longer period via a catheter in the neck. However, experience shows that problems often occur, particularly infections of the catheter or stenoses and occlusions of the veins in the chest caused by the catheter. As a result, the catheter must then be removed and a new catheter inserted via the other side of the neck or, in rare cases, via the groin. The durability of catheters is significantly lower than that of shunts, even though the latter can sometimes become occluded. Therefore, it can be said that blood purification should only be performed permanently via a catheter in exceptional cases.

130. ***Why do some patients have a permanent catheter in the neck?***

Even though dialysis via a catheter, which is inserted through a neck vein and advanced into the right atrium, should be kept as brief as possible or avoided altogether, this is not always possible. For example, if a kidney transplant from a living donor is planned, it may make sense to perform dialysis temporarily via a catheter instead of creating a shunt. Older patients with poor vessels and therefore a high risk that a shunt will not function also often benefit from a catheter. This is especially true if the estimated remaining life expectancy is only a few weeks or months.

Another situation in which a catheter is often placed and dialysis is performed via it is sudden (i.e., acute) kidney dysfunction or kidney failure. In these cases, blood purification is only temporarily necessary, so the more complex surgical creation of a shunt is usually not performed.

In cases of long-term dialysis dependency, a shunt should be created and used for dialysis whenever possible.

Vascular Injuries Caused by Accidents

131. ***As a first responder at the scene of an accident, should you apply a tourniquet to the leg if it is bleeding heavily?***

In principle, any spurting bleeding should be stopped by compression. This can be achieved by applying direct pressure with the hand or fist, but also by using a tourniquet with an object, such as a cloth or belt. It is important, however, that the tourniquet is applied above the source of bleeding in order to cut off blood flow to the site of the vascular injury. Since skin and tissue injuries can also occur at the site of the tourniquet, the pressure applied should not be too great and the tourniquet should not be left in place longer than necessary. Rather, rapid transport to a hospital is extremely important so that the injury can be treated as quickly as possible.

132. ***Can every vascular injury be recognized by heavy bleeding?***

Active, spurting bleeding is certainly the most striking sign of a vascular injury. However, not every injury to an artery is externally visible as bleeding. This may be because only the inner wall of the vessel is torn, while the outer wall remains intact. In such cases, there is no significant bleeding. However, there is a high risk that the vessel will become occluded, resulting in impaired blood flow. Even if the vessel is completely severed, bleeding is not necessarily visible externally. This is because the severed ends of the vessel can retract and thus prevent bleeding from the vessel stump. This ability of severed arteries to roll up is a protective mechanism of the body to prevent exsanguination.

133. ***Are vascular injuries common?***

Minor vascular injuries are very common; strictly speaking, every bleeding skin wound involves injury to a vessel. Serious vascular injuries are rare, as the larger vessels are not superficial but are always protected beneath the muscles. Nevertheless, major trauma, such as from accidents or physical altercations, can

S. Regus, *Answering Patients' Questions About Vascular Medicine*,
https://doi.org/10.1007/978-3-662-72771-3_11

result in injuries to arteries. These are most often injuries to the arms or legs, and less commonly to the neck, chest, or abdominal area. The larger the injured vessel, the more severe and dangerous the bleeding can be, which can ultimately be life-threatening.

134. ***When do vascular injuries occur?***

There are various causes of vascular injuries. Most commonly, these are accidents, especially traffic and sports accidents. Violent altercations can also lead to injuries of arteries or veins. Here, injuries caused by sharp or pointed objects are particularly noteworthy, but massive force resulting in bone fractures or joint dislocations can also be a cause. Finally, medical procedures can also cause vascular injuries, especially needle punctures for diagnostic purposes. The most common example is the so-called cardiac catheterization, in which the coronary arteries are examined and, if necessary, dilated or treated with a stent. To access the coronary arteries, the femoral or radial artery is most commonly punctured. The puncture sites must then be compressed, as otherwise bleeding or rebleeding may occur.

135. ***Can you bleed to death from a vascular injury?***

A vascular injury can lead to occlusion of the artery, resulting in impaired blood flow to the hand (in the case of arm injuries) or foot (in the case of leg injuries). This manifests as pain, a sensation of cold, and numbness. There can also be spurting bleeding from the vessel, which can lead to significant blood loss within a very short time. In extreme cases, it is possible to bleed to death from a vascular injury, especially if a large vessel is involved. In severely injured patients who die at the scene of an accident, the cause is often injuries to the chest or abdominal area, leading to bleeding from the large main artery (aorta). This can result in massive blood loss of several liters within seconds, causing instantaneous death at the scene. Injuries to the arteries of the extremities, i.e., the arm or leg, rarely result in death from exsanguination, especially since these bleedings are externally visible and can at least temporarily be stopped by applying pressure.

136. ***Is it possible that an amputation becomes necessary after a vascular injury?***

After a severe injury, such as a completely dislocated knee or elbow joint, there can be a complete tear of arteries and veins. Often, it is initially possible to suture these vessels back together. However, this usually requires interposing veins. In some cases, however, the tissue damage is so extensive that amputation is necessary from the outset.

In some patients, even after successful reconstruction of the vessels, it may subsequently become necessary to perform an amputation. This is particularly the case if the circulatory disturbance has persisted for several hours and the tissue damage has become too great as a result. After blood flow is restored, the tissue damage can even worsen, as the reintroduction of oxygen leads to the formation of so-called radicals in the tissue, causing additional injury. This tissue damage is associated with increasing tension and swelling, known as compartment syndrome. The waste products released from the damaged tissue into the bloodstream can cause severe harm to the body, with serious effects on the heart, kidneys, and brain. In such cases, amputation must be performed to save the patient's life.

137. ***Is it true that trauma surgeons treat vascular injuries after accidents?***

In principle, trauma surgeons are the specialists for all accident-related injuries. This includes, above all, bone fractures, but also injuries to smaller vessels. However, when larger vessels are injured, vascular surgeons are responsible. Therefore, vascular injuries following accidents—medically referred to as traumatic vascular injuries—are almost always managed in collaboration between vascular and trauma surgery.

138. ***Can athletes protect themselves from vascular injuries?***

Since vascular injuries in athletes result from accidents or overuse, they can be avoided by steering clear of dangerous situations and excessive strain. However, 100% protection does not exist. Especially in high-risk sports, which may involve being at high altitudes, risk of falling, high speeds, and risk of crashing, injuries to arteries and veins can still occur, potentially leading to life-threatening situations. Appropriate protective equipment is definitely recommended and can prevent the majority of injuries or at least reduce their severity, but even then, complete protection cannot be guaranteed.

139. ***Is it necessary to take blood thinners after vascular surgery due to an injury?***

Blood thinning with a so-called platelet inhibitor (medically: antiplatelet agent) is generally necessary when operating on calcified vessels. The reason for this is that blood coagulation is increased in calcified vessels, leading to the formation of clots. These clots can completely block the vessel or be carried further downstream. In such cases, a sudden vessel occlusion occurs, which can cause severe pain and a sensation of coldness. The calcifications are the underlying cause of the arterial narrowings in these cases.

In cases of vascular injuries caused by trauma, it is usually healthy and non-calcified arteries that are affected. Here, blood thinning is fundamentally not necessary, although it may be required for several weeks or a few months after surgery and restoration of the vessel. This is because the inner wall of the vessel at the suture sites is altered by the operation, making clot formation more likely. These irregularities are generally smoothed out again after 6–10 weeks, and blood thinning is then no longer necessary.

140. ***What happens if, in addition to vessels, nerves are also injured in the accident?***

Artery, vein, and nerve usually lie next to each other within a common loose sheath, the so-called neurovascular bundle. Therefore, especially in the area of joints, a dislocation (medically: joint luxation) can result in injury to all three structures. The mechanism of injury in these cases is overstretching of the structures, which may eventually partially or completely tear. However, since nerves are significantly more elastic than the adjacent vessels, it is not uncommon to observe that they are the only one of the three structures to remain intact. If, however, the nerves are also severed, they should be sutured whenever possible. Nevertheless, functional deficits after such nerve suturing are still noticeable: there will be loss of sensation as well as impaired movement of individual muscles until the nerve ends have properly grown back together. This can take several weeks or even months. In addition, it is possible that function remains permanently impaired. However, it is certain that there will be a permanent disturbance of mobility and sensation if the nerves are not sutured and the ends are so far apart that regrowth is not possible. Therefore, every effort should be made to approximate the nerve ends and connect them so that they can grow back together over time. This provides the best conditions for functional recovery.

Vascular Diseases in Athletes

141. ***Can healthy young athletes develop vascular diseases?***

The majority of vascular diseases arise due to vascular calcification, or arteriosclerosis. Risk factors for these vascular diseases include smoking, high blood pressure, elevated blood lipids, overweight and lack of physical activity, as well as diabetes. Since athletes generally do not, or only rarely, exhibit these risk factors, they usually do not suffer from vascular calcification. However, athletes can also develop vascular diseases. These include, for example, vascular injuries following falls or accidents, which are typically acute, meaning they occur suddenly and are often associated with severe bleeding.

Vascular diseases in athletes can also develop as a result of extraordinary physical strain over many years. For example, professional cyclists are at risk of developing narrowing of the iliac artery due to the constant flexion and extension at the hip joint and the aerodynamic position. The technical term for this is "iliac endofibrosis," where "iliac" refers to the pelvic arteries, "endo" means inner, and "fibrosis" stands for hardening. This leads to a thickening of the inner layer of the iliac artery and, as a result, to a narrowing or even occlusion of the artery.

142. ***How do athletes notice that they have vascular problems?***

Patients with vascular calcification (atherosclerosis) notice their vascular problems by the fact that they can walk increasingly shorter distances, i.e., they suffer from intermittent claudication. Typically, they have to stop after walking a certain distance, take a short break, and can then continue walking. To make this waiting period as inconspicuous as possible, many patients look into shop windows, which is where the term "shop window disease" comes from. Open sores on the feet that no longer heal can also be signs of vascular calcification.

S. Regus, *Answering Patients' Questions About Vascular Medicine*,
https://doi.org/10.1007/978-3-662-72771-3_12

In athletes, it is usually the case that they have no complaints in everyday life, but only notice symptoms during physical exertion in training or during maximum effort in competition. Here, too, pain typically occurs in the muscles, which disappears at rest and with normal activity. Since there are many causes for such muscle pain, which are also more likely in athletes than vascular narrowing, making the correct diagnosis is often difficult and is frequently made only many years later.

143. ***Is painful tension in the lower legs during sports a vascular disease?***

Painful tension in the lower legs that occurs under exertion, especially during sports, can have many causes. Among others, a vascular disease may be underlying, which is why blood flow measurements and a consultation with a vascular specialist should be arranged.

However, it is much more likely that diseases of the muscles are the cause, leading to tension in the muscle sheaths. This is referred to as compartment syndrome, where "compartment" means muscle groups enclosed by firm sheaths. Further diagnostics in suspected compartment syndrome particularly include pressure measurement in the tissue, which is performed with special measuring devices.

144. ***Which vessels are most commonly affected in athletes?***

In principle, all vessels can be injured in athletes, although there are particularly vulnerable regions here as well. In cases of **sudden vascular injuries** following accidents, the arteries that are more superficial or run near bones and joints are most often affected. Direct injuries from sharp or pointed objects are rare; more commonly, vessels are torn or ruptured following joint and bone injuries.

In **chronic** vascular injuries, i.e., those developing over a longer period, the vessels located near joints are particularly at risk. This is because the greatest stress occurs here during movement. In cyclists, for example, the iliac artery is typically affected, as it is especially stressed by the aerodynamic position (leaning forward) and the constant high-frequency pedaling. In long-distance runners, the femoral artery can be particularly affected, and otherwise, the popliteal artery is also typically involved in sports-related diseases.

145. ***How are vascular diseases in athletes treated?***

Depending on which vessels are affected, purely conservative therapy with pain medication, cessation of activity, and immobilization may be sufficient. In some cases, however, it may be necessary to switch sports or even to stop the professional practice of a particular sport that is causing the problem (for example, in the case of a cyclist).

It may also be necessary to suture or replace the injured vessel if it has been severed in an accident or is occluded due to chronic stress.

Since every operation also carries risks, the indication for surgery should be made with strict criteria. The decisive factors are always the patient's specific problem and their individual level of suffering.

146. ***Which sports are most frequently affected by vascular diseases?***

Sports in which a specific movement is performed regularly, such as cycling, long-distance running, or cross-country skiing, are most frequently affected by vascular diseases. This can be explained by the fact that the constant repetitive movement, for example, the rapid pedaling and flexion and extension at the hip joint in cycling, causes pressure and shear stress on the iliac arteries. After years of training and competition, this can lead to narrowing or occlusion of these arteries.

Sudden vascular injuries can occur in any sport, especially where there is a high risk of injury. This includes, for example, team sports such as handball, soccer, or basketball, as well as sports with a high risk of falls and resulting injuries.

147. ***What is meant by "cyclist's disease"?***

The so-called cyclist's disease refers to narrowing of the iliac arteries. The condition is also known as **iliac endofibrosis,** where "iliac" stands for pelvis and "endo" for the inner layer of the artery. "Fibrosis" describes a thickening and hardening of the vessel wall. The external iliac artery, medically referred to as the arteria iliaca externa, is particularly affected. This artery branches from the common iliac artery (arteria iliaca communis) and is also flexed with every movement at the hip joint. This causes mechanical stress on the artery, which can lead to small tears in the vessel wall and injuries. After many years of intensive training, this can result in narrowing and occlusion of the iliac artery. This can cause typical problems, especially a feeling of weakness in the affected leg during exertion and in competition. Patients often report muscle pain, also known as ischemic pain, with the left leg being affected significantly more often than the right.[1]

148. ***Can vascular diseases in athletes regress if a break from sports is taken?***

In the vast majority of cases, symptoms during exertion can be reduced or disappear entirely, which, however, means that the athlete must refrain from the triggering sport. This can pose particular difficulties for professional cyclists or long-distance triathletes, as they earn their living through sport. In such cases, the level of suffering is usually very high and the willingness to give up the sport is very low. This may be an indication to initiate and perform a surgical intervention. In this procedure, the narrowed artery is opened, the hardened and thickened vessel wall causing the narrowing is removed, and a patch is sewn in to widen the vessel. In some cases, it may also be necessary to sew in what is known as an interposition graft. This means that the diseased section of the vessel is removed and replaced with a tubular vascular substitute.[2]

---

[1] Regus, S. (2021). Iliac endofibrosis in cyclists and triathletes. essentials. Springer, Wiesbaden. https://doi.org/10.1007/978-3-658-33433-8.

[2] Regus, S. (2021). Therapy options. In: Iliac endofibrosis in cyclists and triathletes. essentials. Springer, Wiesbaden. https://doi.org/10.1007/978-3-658-33433-8_4.

A regression of vascular stenoses is not possible in the vast majority of cases, even with a break from sports.

149. ***Whom should an athlete contact if they suspect a vascular disease?***

Most athletes are highly aware of even the slightest changes in their own performance and, if symptoms arise, will research possible causes. However, treating sports physicians and physiotherapists would also be possible contacts to investigate the cause. If the described symptoms are generally consistent with a vascular disease, it is advisable to consult a vascular specialist. This includes angiologists and vascular surgeons, who deal with all types of vascular diseases on a daily basis. However, if further measures, especially surgery, become necessary, it is advisable to seek care at a treatment center. It is particularly important that sports-related diseases are treated regularly there, as these are overall very rare and complex vascular conditions.

150. ***Are there treatment centers in Germany that specialize in vascular diseases in athletes?***

Currently, there is no treatment center for sports-associated vascular diseases, although such a center would certainly be sensible and necessary. Depending on the affected body and vascular region, specialists with the relevant expertise in treatment can be sought. Typical keywords would be, for example:

- **iliac endofibrosis** for the "cyclist's disease" of the pelvic arteries
- **popliteal entrapment syndrome** for diseases of the popliteal artery
- **adductor canal syndrome** for stenoses of the femoral artery
- **thoracic outlet syndrome** for stenoses of the subclavian artery
- **exercise-induced compartment syndrome** for sensations of tightness and hardening of the calf during and after exertion

Varicose Veins

151. ***Are varicose veins called that because they cause cramps?***

The term "varicose veins" does not, as is often mistakenly assumed, derive from the word "cramp", but rather from the Middle German word "krump". This translates roughly as "crooked" or "winding". Varicose veins are superficial veins that are typically dilated due to leaky venous valves, causing them to become tortuous (see Fig. 1). Although varicose veins can also lead to calf cramps, the most common symptoms are evening swelling of the legs and the visibly tortuous and thickened veins.

152. ***Are varicose veins the most common vascular disease?***

Varicose veins are a very common vascular disease, affecting about one in five people over the course of their lives. Changes in the veins, including so-called spider veins or varicose veins that are not yet visible externally, affect approximately 80% of the adult population, with women being somewhat more frequently affected than men. Even though varicose veins are very common and many people develop them during their lifetime, they are a harmless and usually easily treatable vascular disease. Life-threatening situations, whether during conservative or surgical therapy, are extremely rare.

153. ***Are varicose veins inherited?***

There is indeed an inherited form of varicose veins that appears at birth or in early childhood. However, these hereditary diseases are extremely rare. Acquired varicose veins, which develop over the course of life, are much more common. Risk factors include previous or past thromboses, predominantly standing or sitting occupations, pregnancies, and overweight. It is not uncommon, however, to observe a familial clustering of varicose veins, which could indicate a certain genetic predisposition. Nevertheless, varicose veins are a widespread condition that is primarily caused by our upright posture and the resulting strain on the venous system.

S. Regus, *Answering Patients' Questions About Vascular Medicine*,
https://doi.org/10.1007/978-3-662-72771-3_13

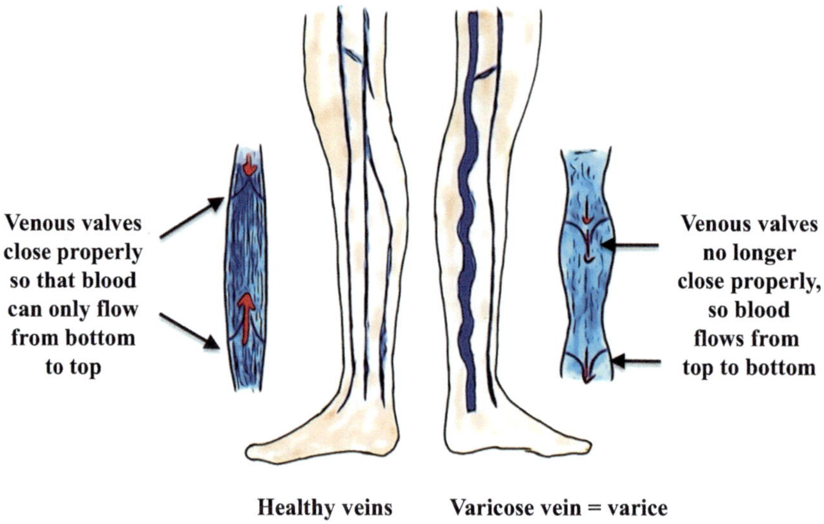

Fig. 1 Difference between healthy veins with functional venous valves and varicose veins with "leaky" valves, in which the blood flows from top to bottom following gravity

154. ***Why do so many women develop varicose veins during pregnancy?***

During pregnancy, the pressure in the abdominal cavity increases due to the steadily growing fetus, which makes it more difficult for venous blood to return to the heart. This leads to congestion of venous outflow, which can promote the development of varicose veins. Deep vein thromboses can also occur during pregnancy and may ultimately trigger varicose vein disease. In addition, hormonal factors play a role, as pregnancy typically leads to a loosening of connective tissue, reducing the stability and elasticity (stretchability) of the veins. This is also a risk factor for the development of varicose veins.

155. ***What is the difference between vascular surgeons and phlebologists?***

Vascular surgeons treat all vascular diseases, especially those of high-pressure vessels (arteries), but also those from the low-pressure system (veins). Vascular diseases of the arteries include stenoses (narrowings in peripheral arterial disease), which lead to circulatory disorders, as well as aneurysms (dilations), which can rupture in the worst case. Diseases of the low-pressure system include thromboses and varicose veins, which are treated by both vascular surgeons and phlebologists. Since arterial diseases are often complex and require elaborate care, and are associated with a higher risk of bleeding, these operations are usually performed in hospitals under inpatient conditions.

Venous diseases, on the other hand, the specialty of phlebologists, are generally treated on an outpatient basis in the office, both conservatively and surgically.

156. ***Why aren't all varicose veins operated on?***

In principle, varicose veins can be treated with compression therapy without surgery. This is possible for all forms of varicose veins except for a few exceptions, such as clot formation in the varicose vein with pronounced inflammation and pus accumulation. Furthermore, varicose veins can be treated from the inside (medically endovenous) using heat (laser or radio waves) or sclerosing solutions or foams (sclerotherapy). For this, the sclerosing agents must be injected into the varicose vein, or the heat applied to the inner wall via catheters inserted into the vein. Finally, the diseased varicose vein can also be removed surgically.

Ultimately, it is the patient who decides whether and especially how their varicose veins are treated or not. The advantage of surgery is that the dilated superficial veins are removed, and no further reflux can occur through them. Wearing a medical compression stocking is then only necessary for a few days at most. This is a significant advantage for patients who find wearing the stocking uncomfortable. The disadvantage of surgery is that, even with the smallest procedure, there are possible risks and complications. These include, for example, bleeding or rebleeding, the formation of large hematomas, and injury to nerves or arteries. Nerve injury can lead to sensory loss and pain in the leg, while injury to arteries can cause significant bleeding. Therefore, the most suitable procedure should be selected for each patient. The patient decides after being thoroughly informed by the treating physicians.

157. ***What catheter procedures are available?***

There are various catheter-based procedures used to treat varicose veins. What they all have in common is that the affected vein is punctured from the outside with a very fine needle, after which a catheter is inserted. Through this catheter, the diseased vein can be closed "from the inside". The main types are:

- Laser procedure (Endovenous Laser Therapy, EVLT):
  In this method, the vein is heated with laser energy. This causes the vein walls to shrink and permanently stick together.
- Radiofrequency procedure (RFO):
  The principle is similar to that of the laser. Instead of laser light, radio waves are used, which also generate heat and thus close the vein.
- Foam or liquid sclerotherapy:
  In this method, a special sclerosing agent is introduced directly into the vein via the catheter. This irritates the vein wall, causing it to become inflamed, stick together, and eventually close permanently. This method is particularly suitable for smaller veins.

All these procedures have in common that the vein remains in the body but is closed from the inside. Over time, it transforms into a fibrous cord.

158. ***What is special about catheter-based procedures?***

The special feature of catheter-based procedures is that, in most cases, no (or at most a small) skin incision is necessary, since in the majority of cases the vein to be treated can be punctured from the outside with a needle. Through this, the catheter, which has a probe at its tip, is inserted into the varicose vein. The vein is then sclerosed from the inside using heat or laser applications, causing the vein walls to stick together. This in turn leads to closure of the dilated vein, which over the next weeks and months transforms into a fibrous cord. In this procedure, the vein is not removed, but is induced to close. The result is the same as if the vein were completely removed, but the approach is gentler. However, catheter-based procedures also carry risks; among other things, burns to the skin can occur, as the veins are usually in direct contact with the skin surface. For this reason, a fluid is infiltrated around the vein during catheter-based procedures, which also contains a local anesthetic. This results in significantly less pain and also reduces the risk of skin burns.

159. ***Which varicose veins can be sclerosed?***

A wide variety of varicose veins can be closed by catheter-based procedures and sclerosing agents that cause the vein walls to stick together. In particular, smaller and deeper varicose veins can often be successfully treated in this way. Large varicose veins located directly under the skin have the disadvantage that sclerosing agents and heat or laser applications in catheter-based procedures can cause burns to the skin. In the case of particularly large varicose veins, the use of heat is often not successful. Therefore, treatment in several steps is usually necessary in these cases, or a surgical approach is recommended. Thanks to advances in science and technology, the available devices have become increasingly sophisticated, making it possible to use endovenous catheter-based procedures even for very large varicose veins. As a result, varicose veins are being treated with catheter-based procedures more and more frequently in recent years. This trend is expected to continue.

160. ***When are stockings alone sufficient as therapy?***

In principle, almost all venous diseases can be treated with compression therapy. Surgery is only recommended if compression stockings are not tolerated or cannot be worn permanently. In the case of very large varicose veins that become inflamed regularly and cause problems, surgery may also become unavoidable. In addition, chronic varicose veins can place a burden on the deep venous system, which can ultimately worsen the problem.

161. ***How is compression therapy performed?***

In compression therapy, consistent wearing of stockings or application of compression bandages is essential, as this is the only way to achieve effective therapy and prevent further complications of varicose veins. This refers to wearing medical compression stockings or elastic compression bandaging with wraps. The advantage of compression by wrapping is that putting on and taking off compression stockings is not required. Depending on the patient's constitution and physical condition, putting on compression stockings can sometimes be quite difficult. For this reason, there are aids available for putting them on; taking them off is generally easier and usually possible without special aids. Removing compression bandages is even easier. However, the disadvantage of compression by elastic wrapping is that the pressure generated by the wrapping is not constant and can vary. It depends on who applies the wrap. Assistance is always required, ideally from a healthcare professional with the necessary expertise and experience in applying compression bandages. The advantage of compression stockings is that, although help is often needed to put them on, the pressure exerted by the stocking is predetermined and constant, depending on the compression class.

162. ***Why aren't my varicose veins operated on, even though their appearance bothers me so much?***

In principle, all forms of varicose veins can be treated surgically. This includes both open and endovenous procedures using laser, radiofrequency, or foam.

However, before any of these so-called invasive procedures, one should be aware that complications can also occur. Especially if the varicose veins do not cause symptoms such as swelling or pain, but are merely a cosmetic issue, this should be taken into account when considering the indication for treatment. Even with small so-called spider veins, problems can arise during treatment. For example, after sclerotherapy, inflammation of the skin and discoloration can occur. In surgical procedures, complications can include wound healing disorders, and in endovenous procedures, inflammation of the treated varicose veins. Therefore, treating physicians may advise against varicose vein surgery if the indication is "only" cosmetic and the risk of complications is increased.

Thromboses

163. ***Are varicose veins and thromboses the same thing?***

Varicose veins and thromboses have in common that they are both venous diseases. However, the two conditions differ fundamentally in several aspects: In thromboses, a clot forms in the vein, which then becomes occluded. Varicose veins, on the other hand, are dilated superficial veins—meaning veins that run directly under the skin—whose venous valves no longer close properly. Venous valves prevent blood in the vein from flowing downward due to gravity. The desired direction of flow in a vein is from bottom to top or from the periphery toward the heart. If, over the years, the vein dilates as a result of aging, the valves can no longer close and essentially fail. As a result, blood flows back and leads to the typical symptoms of congestion in the legs, and sometimes also in the arms. This can be explained by the fact that blood is no longer adequately transported away and accumulates in the tissues. In the early stages, external compression using stockings or compression bandages can help the valves close normally again. In advanced stages, stockings only help to reduce the symptoms of congestion; the valve function can no longer be restored. In such cases, if the patient is significantly affected, only surgery—by removing or sclerosing the varicose veins—can provide relief.

Thromboses are treated conservatively in the majority of cases, that is, with blood thinning and compression therapy using stockings or compression bandages. Only in selected cases can clots be removed surgically.

164. ***My leg is often swollen in the evening—is this a thrombosis?***

Evening swelling of the leg can be due to blood congestion. This is especially the case after prolonged standing or sitting, as gravity can cause blood to pool. This is particularly true for varicose veins, since the bulging of the veins means the venous valves no longer close properly, allowing blood to flow back downward due to gravity. Therefore, varicose vein disease is one of the most common causes

S. Regus, *Answering Patients' Questions About Vascular Medicine*,
https://doi.org/10.1007/978-3-662-72771-3_14

of evening leg swelling. Thrombosis of the leg veins can also cause leg swelling, but in this case, the swelling is present during the day as well and does not only occur after prolonged standing or sitting.

Another cause of evening leg swelling can be heart failure, which typically leads to swelling of the lower legs and feet in the evening, with the swelling subsiding by the next morning. In addition, there is often increased nighttime urination, as the blood that has accumulated in the legs during the day is more easily transported back to the heart when lying down and then excreted by the kidneys.

165. ***Are thromboses more common than arterial diseases?***

Venous thromboses are the most common venous disease, with the likelihood of developing the condition increasing with age. The leg veins are particularly affected, as blood can more easily "pool" in the upright human. The risk of developing a thrombosis increases with age: among children, one in 100,000 is affected; among 40-year-olds, about 0.1%, and among those over 70, about 1–2% suffer from thrombosis of the deep venous system.

The most common arterial disease is peripheral arterial occlusive disease, abbreviated as PAOD. Here, too, there is a marked increase with age. The likelihood of disease is low in children. At age 40, about 1–2% are affected, and from age 70, the likelihood rises to about 15–20%.

Thus, in Germany, more people are affected by PAOD, the most common arterial disease, than by venous thromboses. Both conditions increase in frequency over the course of life. In peripheral arterial occlusive disease, risk factors such as high blood pressure, smoking, and lack of exercise play a major role. It is therefore to be expected that the number of cases will continue to rise in the coming years.

166. ***Why do female smokers who take the birth control pill have a higher risk of thrombosis?***

Both smoking (in particular, the ingredients in cigarettes such as tar and nicotine) and the hormones contained in contraceptives (commonly referred to as the "pill") have an effect on blood coagulation. More precisely, they increase the tendency for blood to clot, thereby raising the risk of thrombosis. In addition, they can cause narrowing and inflammation of blood vessel walls. This affects both arteries and, in particular, veins. Smoking and the pill each increase the risk of thrombosis on their own, but the combination of smoking and the pill leads to a tenfold increase in thrombosis risk. Therefore, patients should be informed about this risk and, ideally, should refrain from smoking (also referred to as nicotine abuse).

Incidentally, the same effect occurs with smoking hashish, which has become a topic of discussion following the legalization of cannabis. However, cannabis primarily affects the red blood cells; specifically, the red blood cells swell immediately after smoking hashish. The longer and more frequently someone uses cannabis, the more pronounced this effect becomes. Therefore, women who take contraceptives should also be informed about the side effects and the increased risk of thrombosis associated with hashish use.

167. ***Can a thrombosis be detected by blood tests?***

In the case of thrombosis, blood values are typically altered, especially the so-called D-dimer value. However, this value is not specific for thrombosis, meaning it can also be elevated in other diseases and conditions. Therefore, blood values alone are not sufficient to detect a thrombosis. Much more important are the symptoms reported by the patient, the physical examination findings, and ultrasound. Conversely, a D-dimer value within the normal range makes thrombosis unlikely. For this reason, the D-dimer value is always determined in blood tests when ruling out or confirming a thrombosis.

168. ***When does a thrombosis need to be operated on?***

In most cases, a thrombosis can be treated conservatively. This includes compression and blood thinning. These measures usually reduce or eliminate the symptoms of thrombosis and prevent further clot formation. Blood thinning is usually necessary for 3–6 months, whereas compression therapy, which is performed using bandages and medical stockings, should generally be continued for a longer period (1–2 years). Compression therapy can reduce long-term symptoms and complications that arise after thrombosis. These include, for example, chronic swelling and open sores on the legs. In such cases, surgery may be necessary to reopen the occluded veins and improve outflow. Short-segment thromboses of the pelvic veins, especially in young women, can also be a reason for surgery. These thromboses in the pelvic area can be caused by narrowing of the left pelvic vein, which results from its crossing with the pelvic artery. This condition is known as May-Thurner syndrome, named after its original describers.

169. ***How great is the risk that I will get another thrombosis after having one?***

Anyone who has previously suffered from thrombosis has a higher risk of developing it again. This is partly because the existing thrombosis has already caused some damage. Even if the thrombosis has resolved over time, changes to the vein wall are typical and lead to an increased risk of thrombosis. In addition, coagulation disorders that originally caused the thrombosis may be present, further increasing the overall risk of thrombosis. Therefore, it is recommended to have a coagulation test performed after a second episode of thrombosis. If a coagulation disorder is confirmed, long-term anticoagulation may become necessary. This is required in such cases to prevent the risk of a severe thrombosis.

170. ***Can thrombosis injections prevent a thrombosis before a long flight?***

During a long flight (the same applies to long car journeys), the risk of thrombosis is increased. This is because movement is restricted and blood can more easily "pool" in the legs. Regular breaks and getting up during the flight can help. Compression stockings can also be worn on the plane or during car travel. For people who have some pre-existing damage or have already had a thrombosis, a so-called thrombosis injection may be recommended. These are anticoagulant medications, which are also administered in cases of acute thrombosis. They are injected once or twice daily into the subcutaneous fat tissue and prevent further extension of the thrombosis while supporting the dissolution of clots. Therefore, in certain situations, such as before a flight, it may make sense to administer a thrombosis injection beforehand. If in doubt, it is advisable to discuss this with your treating physician, usually your general practitioner.

171. ***Can you die from a thrombosis?***

Thrombosis itself is not considered life-threatening, but complications can occur. The most severe and sometimes life-threatening complication is pulmonary embolism. In this case, clots from the thrombosis are carried to the lungs and block large vessels, which can lead to shortness of breath and even circulatory collapse. Therefore, thrombosis—even if it involves smaller veins in the leg—should be treated as a serious condition and requires medical supervision. Compression therapy and the administration of anticoagulant medications are important. Both measures can reduce the risk of fatal complications, so fortunately, fatal complications from thrombosis are extremely rare today.

172. ***How long do I need to take anticoagulants for a thrombosis?***

The duration of anticoagulant medication for thrombosis depends on the extent and location of the clot formation. For superficial vein thrombosis (referred to as thrombophlebitis), 2–6 weeks may be sufficient. For deep vein thrombosis, usually in the leg, anticoagulant therapy is generally recommended for 3–6 months. If multiple thromboses have already occurred, lifelong "blood thinning" may be necessary. This is especially the case if certain conditions are present that increase the risk of clotting. Various factors of the blood coagulation system may be affected. All conditions associated with increased blood clotting are referred to as thrombophilia. In cases of thrombophilia, long-term medication is usually necessary to reduce the blood's ability to clot and thus prevent thrombosis.

GPSR Compliance

The European Union's (EU) General Product Safety Regulation (GPSR) is a set of rules that requires consumer products to be safe and our obligations to ensure this.

If you have any concerns about our products, you can contact us on ProductSafety@springernature.com

In case Publisher is established outside the EU, the EU authorized representative is:

Springer Nature Customer Service Center GmbH
Europaplatz 3
69115 Heidelberg, Germany

Batch number: 10739795

Printed by Printforce, the Netherlands